WHITE STOCKINGS, CAPS and STARCH

WHITE STOCKINGS, CAPS *and* STARCH

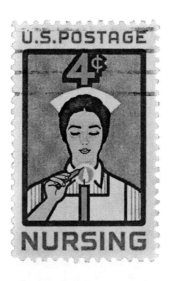

Carolyn Ukura Kuechle

Jan Kmieciak Stenson

MILL CITY PRESS

Mill City Press, Inc.
322 First Avenue N, 5th floor
Minneapolis, MN 55401
612.455.2293
www.millcitypublishing.com

The front cover depicts a student nurse lighting a candle portraying the passing of the flame from Florence Nightengale. The flame symbolized dedication to caring for patient needs. This stamp was issued in 1961 commemorating one hundred years of nurse education in the United States. It has special meaning to our class since it was the year we entered Methodist Hospital School of Nursing.

ISBN-13: 978-1-62652-118-6
LCCN: 2014904751

Cover Design by Mary Ross
Typeset by Kristeen Ott

Printed in the United States of America

We dedicate this writing to all nurses,

including those who came before, and

all who will come after us.

May they always have great compassion

for those in their care.

"a glimpse of the

way the were."

To Mary

Carolyn Ylura Kuechle

INTRODUCTION

The three-year hospital-based diploma nursing school is the oldest traditional nursing school in the United States. Today very few diploma schools remain. The "convent-like" style of living that we experienced beginning in 1961 at Methodist Hospital in Saint Louis Park, Minnesota, seems worthy of being remembered. Therefore, this writing.

This was a unique experience where we lived together in the dormitory adjacent to the hospital. We attended classes in the hospital basement nursing school. During our freshman year, we rode the orange school bus for our in-depth science classes at Augsburg College. The hospital provided our area of practice in learning "hands-on" patient care and nursing procedures with our instructors by our side. And, during our working for pay shifts, we had the opportunity of learning on our own.

This writing began in 2009 with the 1963 Juneau, Alaska, summer working experience of classmates Betty Beard, Vera Kemp, Carolyn Ukura, and Karen Young. Next to be written was chapter one, Waiting for the Bus. After that, the writing became a collaboration between Carolyn Ukura Kuechle and Jan Kmieciak Stenson. Materials used for reference were from memory, in particular, Jan's very excellent memory! We also found our classmate's journaling, diaries, saved schedules, old textbooks, and papers from that time to be invaluable. *Methodist Hospital: A Tradition of Caring* and the *Merck Manual* also aided us in this endeavor.

Most chapters are a collaboration of the two main authors, but when information is primarily from one author, she becomes the chapter author. In that case, her name is noted at the chapter beginning. Other classmates have given information and written stories that have greatly enhanced this writing. Where there are quotes, the author's name is written at the end of the quote.

ACKNOWLEDGMENTS

Classmates Judy Mishek Adams, Mary Peterson Cady, Monyne Jahnke Cotton, Vera Kemp Germain, Karen Young Miller, Velma Jean Shelton, Sue Tingerthal Shull, Vicki Lymburner Thompson, Sandy Johnson Clift Ware, and Betty Beard Welke have written stories and memories, or have provided photos and reference materials.

Larry Kuechle has been there to constantly provide much needed tech support and preparation of the photos and visual aides.

Sharon Ukura Waisanen read the text and made helpful recommendations and improvements.

Jodie Ukura Mirsch RN, offered current hospital information.

Kathy Spence Johnson, MLIS, archivist, Saint Louis Park Historical Society, gave the reference book, *Methodist Hospital: A Tradition of Caring*, by Bill Beck, 1992.

Douglas Crawford-Parker, Shannon Barry Stenson, Jean A. Gardner, and John Helberg helped by giving suggestions and reading parts of this manuscript.

We offer Thanks and Gratitude to all of the above!

CONTENTS

PART ONE BEGINNINGS, SEPTEMBER 1961
1   Waiting for the Bus / 1
2   H. Joan Barber / 8
3   The First Day / 12
4   Getting Acquainted and Reality Strikes / 18
5   Augsburg College, First Semester, 1961 / 24
6   The Uniform / 28
7   Basic Nursing / 31
8   Working for Pay / 36
9   Dorm Life and Housemothers / 46
10   The Pink Ladies / 53
11   Second Semester, January 1962 / 56
12   The Capping Ceremony / 59
13   Basic Nursing II / 66
14   Summer Break, June 1962 / 68

PART TWO THE SECOND YEAR, SEPTEMBER 1962
15   Surgery Rotation / 75
16   Medical and Surgical Nursing / 84
17   Northwest to Alaska / 93

PART THREE THE THIRD YEAR, SEPTEMBER 1963
18   Psychiatric Nursing at Hastings State Hospital / 125
19   Obstetrics and Newborn Nursing / 145
20   Pediatric Nursing / 159
21   Love Stories / 170
22   A Different Course Ahead: The Novice / 177

PART ONE

BEGINNINGS, SEPTEMBER 1961

CHAPTER 1

Waiting for the Bus

By: Carolyn Ukura Kuechle

> The birth of all things
> is weak and tender.
> And, therefore we should have eyes
> intent on beginnings.
> —Michel De Montaigne, *Essays*

It was a perfect summer day, that afternoon of June 21, 1961, as a light, warm breeze rippled through the leaves on the tall maples that stood along the Excelsior Boulevard sidewalk in Saint Louis Park, Minnesota. The blue sky had not a cloud, and the birds sang happily while flitting about building nests, while others were bringing food for their already hatched, ever-hungry broods.

Although it was a perfect summer day, and all seemed very right with the world, my anxiety could not be dispelled. I was standing at the city bus stop tightly clutching the bus transfer in my right hand. And, I had already stood there for nearly a half hour after having taken the wrong downtown city bus. My destination, according to the bus driver, was only a few minutes away.

I was dressed in my most appropriate clothing for what I felt was the most important meeting of my life, thus far. This was for a 1:00 p.m. interview with Miss H. Joan Barber at the new Methodist Hospital School of Nursing. Miss Barber was the founder and director of nursing of the three-year diploma school where I hoped to become a nursing student in just a few months, September 1961.

My navy blue dress with red and white horizontal stripes at the midriff, black pumps, and black leather shoulder bag gave me a feeling of being well dressed and professional. I could feel that my cheeks had flushed and had turned a bright pink while I anxiously stood waiting in the sun. I was quite certain that my fine, short hair was looking very windblown, in spite of the hair spray. However, these problems all paled in comparison to my total unhappiness with myself for having taken the wrong bus and putting my dreams in severe jeopardy. After all, I had been living in his city and riding city buses for over a year now, didn't I know anything? And so my mind circled around as I stood waiting for the bus. Really, why hadn't I inquired for directions and just walked the remaining distance to the hospital, but of course, it was too late to even consider that option now.

I checked my watch for the hundredth time. It now read ten minutes to 1:00 p.m.! And still I waited, with no sign of a city bus anywhere around.

A few weeks earlier, a letter had arrived to the apartment at 3033 Portland Avenue South that I shared with my hometown friends. It had been delivered to my room by whichever one of them had collected the mail that day. The letter was in response to my September 1961 application letter to Methodist Hospital School of Nursing.

Each day I had waited and hoped that I would receive a response to my letter to attend the nursing school. Of course, I hoped for a positive response, but if it was a negative response, at least I could refocus my thinking.

On a Saturday morning, Ramona, my roommate, and I were

in the process of cleaning our bedroom. Ramona, having very thorough cleaning tendencies, thought we should move the dresser to clean behind it. When we moved the dresser, a business-sized, white envelope fell to the floor. As I leaned down to pick up the envelope, I saw that it was from Miss H. Joan Barber, director of nursing at Methodist Hospital School of Nursing! I ripped the envelope open to find that Miss Barber had accepted my letter of application, and she was requesting to be called to schedule an interview. There, wedged between the wall and the dresser, this possibly life-changing document had remained hidden while I had watched and waited! It was a good thing that Ramona was a thorough cleaner.

After finding Miss Barber's letter, it was an agonizing wait until Monday when I could phone her to schedule my interview. Promptly on Monday morning at 9:00 a.m., I dialed the Methodist Hospital phone number while on break from my clerk-typist job at Walter Library. The switchboard operator directed my call to Miss Barber's office, while I waited with bated breath to hear Miss Barber's voice. After introducing myself, and upon hearing Miss Barber's very proper but "cheery" sounding voice, I relaxed. I told her that I had received her letter in response to my nursing school application letter and would very much like to come in for an interview.

"Yes," Miss Barber said, "I will be very happy to meet you, Miss Ukura. Would June 21 at 1:00 p.m. work for you to come to my office?"

Would I? I wanted to scream! But, I very calmly told Miss Barber that June 21 at 1:00 p.m. would certainly work very well for me. As I put the phone down, I thought, *Could this possibly be the first step in my life-long dream to become a nurse?*

To become a registered nurse had been my career choice for so long that I really hadn't thought of much else. Of course, in the 1950s and 1960s, there were not a lot of career choices for women. They were mainly nurse, teacher, social worker, librarian, and office worker.

Family role models had influenced my decision to become a nurse, as there were several nurses in my extended family. Two of my great aunts had not had formal nursing education, but they worked as nurses. Around the year 1916, my great aunt, Minnie Carlson Peterson, had been trained to be a practical nurse by Dr. Walters and his nurse wife within their small town of Moose Lake, Minnesota.

Minnie was my greatest and most important role model. She was a tiny, very humble lady who did not want attention drawn to herself. At the time of the 1918 fire in northeast Minnesota, a reporter from the Saint Paul dispatch had named Minnie a heroine of the fire. Minnie was working at the Moose Lake Community Hospital that October 12, 1918, day of this holocaust. She and her sister, my other great aunt, Ida Carlson Olson, had guided a groggy, partially anesthetized patient from the hospital into Moosehead Lake, a few blocks from the hospital. They saved her, as well as their own lives. Minnie did not like the tone of the article, since she certainly did not consider herself to be a heroine. She was just doing her job.

Minnie went about caring for anyone who came to her in need of help. Later, when she was married and had a family, without benefit of electricity, telephone, or running water, Minnie had taken care of patients in her farm home. As well, soon-to-deliver expectant mothers came to stay in her home. She delivered the baby, then took care of mother and child until the mother felt strong enough to return home. This being the 1930s, and the Great Depression, her payment, many times, might be a chicken, a sack of potatoes, or other farm produce, since most people had very little money.

When I was eleven years old, I had a first-hand hospital and nurse experience while in the pediatric ward of Saint Luke's Hospital in Duluth, Minnesota. I had been ill for several days when I went to see my physician, who recommended emergency surgery for what turned out to be a near-burst appendix. After surgery, he ordered frequent, painful penicillin injections into my posterior to prevent infection. The student nurses who administered the injections were always very kind and caring. I was quite intrigued with them, and I observed their every move. The student nurse bustled about the ward wearing her student nurse uniform of a white, starched pinafore over a blue dress, white shoes, and white hose. She had the nursing cap of her school perched on top of her head. The girls on my six-bed ward were given excellent care by the student nurses. As far as my eleven-year-old mind was concerned, the student nurses were next to angels, and I had every intention that one day I would join their ranks.

Another factor that influenced my career choice came from hearing my parents and other people in my rural community speak of the Great Depression that had occurred in the 1930s. Many people of that time were homeless, jobless, and had little money or means of support. The economy was in disarray, unemployment rates across the country were high, and going into debt was deemed worse than the devil himself. "Hoover days" as they spoke of them, had greatly influenced my life. "If you choose nursing as a career, you will always have a job." This was said to me by my elders.

After graduating McGregor High School, I had come to the "big city," along with several of my classmates and friends, to work and experience what we believed to be an "exciting and fun" life! We had been planning this for some time. We were able to find jobs, mainly entry-level office work. We rented a room or an apartment and pooled our resources to pay expenses. My main goal was to save as much money as I could so I could attend school in a year. I was very fortunate to work as a clerk-typist in the acquisitions department in Walter Library at the University of Minnesota with a caring and wonderful group of people. I was very careful with spending my money, and on my $242 per month salary before taxes, I saved $1,200 that year.

It was against this backdrop that I stood waiting for the city bus that was to take me to Methodist Hospital to this most important appointment of my life. However, no city bus had come along.

What had come down the road were two young men around my age of eighteen. They slowed down while going past me to ask if I would like a ride. They had already driven around the block at least twice, and I appeared to ignore them as they drove on by. I had observed, however, that they seemed to be clean cut and friendly in demeanor.

In the distance, once again, I saw the young men approaching. It's very true that I was desperate, but I had an instinctual feeling that they could be trusted and would not cause harm. They slowed their car as they neared, and the young man in the passenger seat again asked:

Would you like a ride?
Can you get me to Methodist Hospital in ten minutes?
Oh sure we can.

The car pulled over to the curb and stopped directly in front of me. I quickly opened the backseat door and hopped into the car. The two were very friendly, and we chatted on the way to the hospital. They seemed eager to help as I explained my urgency to arrive at my hospital appointment. Within five minutes, I was at the entrance to Methodist Hospital. I profusely thanked the two young men, hopped out of the car, and never saw them again.

Upon entering the hospital, I saw the information desk, where two very friendly appearing "Pink Ladies" sat. I inquired and received direction to the nursing school located on the lower hospital level.

After stepping off the elevator, I turned to go down the nursing school corridor. I looked at the wall to my left where the placard of Miss H. Joan Barber, director of nursing, "jumped" out at me.

I took a deep breath and appeared in the doorway of Miss Barber's office. She stood up from her desk, and with both hands on her hips, she straightened her dress over her slim figure. At about five feet, two inches, she was not very tall, but she took full advantage of every quarter inch of her height with her stately, erect posture. I sensed a certain "air" about Miss Barber that seemed to command respect and an "I'm in charge here" attitude. She had a warm, enthusiastic smile, a hearty laugh, and the long curls in her thick, chestnut-colored hair bobbed as she beckoned me to enter.

Miss Barber extended her hand and motioned me to sit in the chair that was facing her desk while she said: "You must be Miss Ukura." As I took her hand, I said: "Yes, I am, and I'm very pleased to meet you, Miss Barber."

I thought to myself, *And you have no idea what it took for me to arrive here on time. If you did, it might well be all over before it has begun.*

CHAPTER 2

H. Joan Barber

In 1959, Hamline University and Methodist Hospital ended the four-year Hamline-Asbury Methodist nursing program. The newly opened Methodist Hospital in Saint Louis Park began planning for a three-year diploma nursing school. Though money was short, they had a need for the practical work provided by on-site student nurses. The Bishop D. Stanley Coors Education Endowment Fund enabled Methodist Hospital to have start-up money for the nursing school. It had been Bishop Coors's interest during his last illness that the new Methodist Hospital have a nursing school.

H. Joan Barber was appointed to be the founder of the three-year diploma nursing school in early 1961. She came to this position from Sister Kenny Rehabilitation Institute in Minneapolis, where she had spent five years as director of nursing services. Previous to Sister Kenny Rehab Institute, H. Joan had administrative experience at Northwestern Hospital in Minneapolis, William Budge Memorial Hospital in Logan, Utah, and the University of Michigan Hospital in Ann Arbor, Michigan.

Miss Barber was from Michigan, and she received her bachelor of arts degree from Hillsdale College, an independent liberal arts college in southern Michigan. She had studied nursing at the University of Michigan Hospital School of Nursing in Ann Arbor, Michigan, and had done advanced work in nursing administration at Western

Reserve University in Cleveland, Ohio.

While a nursing student at the University of Michigan Hospital School of Nursing in Ann Arbor, Miss Barber wrote an article for the prestigious *American Journal of Nursing* (July 1937 issue) entitled, "The Symbol of the Cross as Used in Nursing." In this article, she does a thorough evaluation of the cross and its significance to the nursing profession. She states that many schools of nursing have a variation of the cross in their school pins. One point of many in this article is that the cross stands for unselfish service, and that those who bear it are eager and ready to soothe those who are suffering, regardless of rank in position, color, or creed.

Having only been employed by Methodist Hospital since early 1961, it must have been quite a daunting task for Miss Barber to get a nursing school up and running, and to be able to admit students into the nursing program by September of that year. Unfortunately, records of the nursing school have been lost or destroyed, so we can only speculate on the enormity of the task. She had to hire nursing instructors to aide in the writing of a curriculum and to teach in the nursing school. Since Augsburg College would be affiliated with the nursing school in providing the necessary college courses, she would have had to coordinate between the college and the nursing school. Setting up the physical layout of the school, getting to know the hospital staff, and coordinating with them to pave the way for students would have been a large involvement, no doubt.

Advertising about the school, and most importantly, gaining qualified students, was yet another area where she devoted her expertise. Each applicant to the school had to be interviewed and a determination made regarding her qualification as a possible student. Miss Barber related that grades were not her only criteria, but how well she felt that person would be as a well-rounded and compassionate bedside nurse. Though there were but twenty-two students accepted into the first class, everything about the program was new and untested. It took a fireball like Miss Barber to do the task!

Miss Barber was very dedicated to the student nurses, and she tried very hard to make us into the very best nurses that we could be. She was an inspiring, and oftentimes interesting, lecturer. A comment she made to us in class one day: "Most of you didn't get into this school because of your admission letter, but in spite of it."

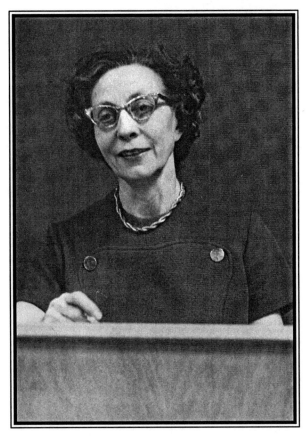

H. Joan Barber

Miss Barber never married, as seemed to be the situation for many professional women of that time. She lived in a little pink house on Vallacher Avenue in Saint Louis Park. She invited us to have our twentieth class reunion at her home in June 1984. On that day, she stood on her little kitchen stool to get to her top kitchen cupboard.

Those of us who watched as she did this just stood there with bated breath. No one admonished her to please stand down. After all, she was still the chief! The curls of her hair no longer bounced as they had in earlier days when she was making a point of elation or agitation. In 1984, her hair was short, straight, and gray.

In 1989, Miss Barber wrote a letter to Karen Young Miller that she could not attend our twenty-fifth class reunion. Her handwriting was very shaky and difficult to read. She wrote:

> I remember your class, and when I think of it,
> I think of the girls in it. I remember your names and
> everything. The other classes I cannot think of the
> names, but your class I know. You weren't so many,
> and I liked you one and all.

H. Joan Barber died in 1991.

The nursing school lasted but fourteen years. In 1975, the last class of forty-four students graduated. The American Nurse's Association and the Citizens Committee for Nursing in Minnesota recommended that hospitals phase out diploma programs in favor of institutions of higher learning within the general system of education. Therefore, two-year community college programs leading to an associate nursing degree became the norm, and it continues today.

We all admired and feared Miss Barber, but we grew to respect her as a very important role model. Her dealings with us were fair and firm. We always felt she would listen to our point of view, and we trusted her. Lifelong advice that Miss Barber gave us: "If you can't change the situation, then you must change your attitude toward it."

CHAPTER 3

The First Day

Monday, September 11, 1961, a sunny, warm, and bright day, twenty-two young women were gathered together for the first time in the Methodist Hospital School of Nursing (MHSN) dormitory lobby. We applied and had been accepted into the first class of the new three-year diploma nursing school. Historically since 1892, Asbury Methodist Hospital had educated registered nurses, beginning with The Asbury Hospital Training School for Nurses. In 1940, the school was affiliated with Hamline University, and it became the Hamline-Asbury Methodist Hospital School of Nursing. However, after nineteen years, the Hamline-Asbury Methodist Hospital School of Nursing ended.

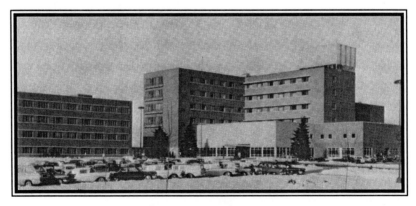

Methodist Hospital, 1960

This was a beginning nursing school program in the newly built 276-bed, six-floor hospital in Saint Louis Park, Minnesota. The hospital had opened in February 1959, after Asbury Methodist Hospital, having served the community very well, became too old and cramped. Asbury Methodist became a long-term care facility until it was sold in 1968.

Within this gathered group of eighteen- and nineteen-year-old women from urban, rural, and small towns of Minnesota and Wisconsin, the largest commonalities we possessed were excitement and apprehension! It was the excitement of beginning to fulfill, for most of us, a long-time dream of becoming professional nurses, and the apprehension of the many unknowns in fulfilling this dream. Three-fourths of the group had graduated high school that spring, and there were many firsts for them. These firsts included living away from home, the first time at college, and the first time of parental independence. The other one-fourth had graduated high school a year earlier and had already experienced the independence of living away and going to college or work.

Most of us entered the dormitory doors that September day in 1961 with much idealism regarding the nursing profession, and our place in it. In short, we probably had no idea what our nursing career would really be like! Some of us knew nursing through the eyes of Cherrie Adams or Sue Barton books, or through TV dramas such as *Dr. Kildare* and *Ben Casey*. Others of us had had close observation of the nurse role while being cared for by nurses as a hospital patient, or by having the nurse role modeled by a close relative.

The lobby was filled that day with people: students, parents, boyfriends, sisters, brothers, and friends. Mountains of suitcases, boxes, stuffed animals, books, shoes, and other items filled any remaining space. We said our goodbyes, and then we faced the reality of being on our own while grappling with a very large question: What is this experience really going to be like, and how will we fit into it?

Thus, we began our journey together, learning, living, and (mostly) loving our profession.

Little did we know that first day that we would form a family that would last fifty years and beyond. Like most families, some of our sisters would stay in close touch, while others would not. Through the years, whenever we were together again, there would be a feeling of familiarity and closeness. We eagerly transported ourselves back in time to our early years in school. Our conversation and our comfort level was as though no time had passed.

As a young girl, the present I remember getting from Santa was a play nurse kit that contained a stethoscope, thermometer, syringe, otoscope, hot water bottle, and an eye chart. I had lots of fun pretending and dreaming of becoming a nurse!

That dream became reality May 5, 1961, after receiving a letter from Miss H. Joan Barber. It stated, "Providing you plan to stay with the program for the full three years, and do the very best you can at all times, we will be most happy to have you in our school." This was exciting news . . . small town girl going to the big city! The matriculation fee of eleven dollars made payable to Methodist Hospital School of Nursing was due before May 30th. Payment to the uniform company for student uniforms and payment for the first semester's tuition was to be paid before we began classes on September 11, 1961.

The morning of September 11, 1961, I filled the 1953 Chevrolet my dad had bought me with my belongings and headed to MHSN. I arrived that morning to settle into home for the next three years. The journey had begun! I thought the hospital, our dorm, and the surrounding area was all beautiful, modern, and very welcoming. Coming from a small high school class, having only twenty-two nursing classmates felt good to me too. I think being the very first class of MHSN, and our being such a small number, bonded special friendships between us . . . a true sisterhood. Miss Barber said, "We know the next three years will be interesting and profitable for you."

She was right! I thought MHSN was a great experience, and I am forever grateful for that opportunity.

—Karen Young Miller

That first day, we each were given our dormitory room number. With our belongings in hand, up to second floor we went. Miss Barber had informed us of whom our roommate would be. Some of us had corresponded, but there were unanswered questions. What would she really be like? Would we become friends, or would living in such close proximity with our roommate become intolerable?

On second floor, we entered a long narrow hall that ran the length of the building with numbered rooms facing the parking lot on the east side of the hallway. Inside were two single beds, two dressers, two desks, two closets, and a sink with a mirror above.

In the center of the long hall was a small booth with two telephones. Little did we know how important these phones would become in keeping us connected with friends and family. (This was a long time before cell phones, iPods, or computers of any kind were available for personal use.) At the south end, the hallway opened up into a lounge area to the west. An exit door onto the balcony was located here, as well. Contained in the lounge were a few "easy" chairs, card tables and chairs, an iron and ironing board, a small TV, and an old storm window that we used to lay our wet, starched caps for stretching and drying.

On the west side of the long hallway was a community bathroom with toilet stalls, bathtubs, showers, sinks, and mirrors. Located next to it was a three-bed room with a spectacular view of a flower garden near the patio below. Beyond that was a view of a natural area, where Meadow Brook meandered through a fresh water swamp and wild flower meadow.

After searching for room numbers, we found and entered our assigned room. Depending upon who arrived first, that person gravitated to the bed by the window. If not already there, our roommate soon arrived, and we met face to face! All fears of who she would be were over, and we began to get acquainted. We unpacked and settled into our space while visiting and learning about each other. After this, we met other classmates, and we discovered our surroundings within the dormitory and in the hospital that was connected to the dormitory.

The four-story dormitory building had three floors of student rooms (second, third, and fourth floors). In 1961, since we were the first class of the new school, only the second floor was being occupied. However, there were some remaining students from the four-year Hamline-Asbury School of Nursing living on third floor, as well as other hospital employees. The first floor was the entry-level floor, and it contained the reception desk, lobby, and elevator. It had a living room with western exposed windows overlooking the natural area. Beyond that, a hallway extended to a small apartment and other bedrooms.

The lower level floor had a kitchen and a large recreation room with a windowed wall looking west to the serene natural wetland. In the foreground were the patio and lawn and a flower garden that we helped tend. At a later time, we realized the focus and ideology of our school director, Miss Barber. It became obvious that her goal was also that we would become well-rounded young women in all areas, not just nursing. Tending a garden was, no doubt, part of her focus.

An entry door to a tunnel was located just off the recreation area. It was used to get into the hospital from the dorm. (This tunnel was also found to be useful for sneaking into the dorm without house-mother knowledge.)

Later that day, we went on a scavenger hunt organized by the outgoing Hamline-Asbury students. The scavenger hunt had a list of items that many of us knew, and others that were totally foreign to most of us. They included: bed pan, thermometer, stethoscope, bandage scissors, tongue blade, IV standard, specimen container, blood pressure cuff, sphygmomanometer, patient gown, and a rubber sheet.

Some of the items were easy to find and identify, and others were very confusing. Having never had much experience with an IV standard, Jan Kmieciak read this item as Roman numerals I and V, meaning the number four. And, she wasn't quite sure what was meant by standard!

CHAPTER 4

Getting Acquainted and Reality Strikes

Food and eating, of course, were always high on our list of importance, including where we could eat for the least amount of money. Our main options were the hospital cafeteria and the coffee shop. Or, as some of us discovered, we could save some money by cooking meals ourselves in the small, downstairs kitchen of the dorm.

What got us into trouble was when we began storing food items in the corners of the dorm room windows, behind the curtains. The food items stayed cooler next to the window, and were very handy for a quick snack. Plus, we didn't have to run down two flights of stairs to the kitchen. This went on for some time until we were absolutely forbidden to have food items stored on the window ledges by the head housemother, Mrs. Nora Boldt. Maybe there were complaints concerning this erroneous behavior, or it was Miss Barber having noticed it. But, the ruling given us by Mrs. Boldt was that this behavior must immediately cease! Perhaps they thought the dorm was beginning to look like a tenement building, or that it totally ruined the image of perfection that was to be portrayed by the nursing school and its student nurses.

The coffee shop was an appealing place to eat. They had wonderful breakfasts, including very delicious cinnamon rolls! There were lots of eggs in the French toast, eggs that overflowed the bread that you could see on your plate when it was served. A fruit plate and toast sprinkled with cinnamon was low cost and tasty. Many "suppers" were eaten there at $1.25 a plate! Mrs. Dibble was the head of the coffee shop, and she was always very kind to the nursing students.

Many meals were eaten in the main cafeteria. The evening cafeteria server gave enough of the meat entrée to share, until the cafeteria supervisor found out and put an abrupt stop to it. Much of the food served there was very good, but they also served some unusual dishes, such as salmon patties with cream sauce and peas with a side of Frito chips. Another oddity that was served was prune whip. Even some of the students enjoyed the unusual dishes. As an example, Jan Kmieciak said, "I tried it, liked it, and ate it fairly often until a patient I was caring for ate his prune whip, and then threw it all up!"

Purchasing meals took a fair amount of our earnings, with little money left at the end of the month. Two students told of pooling their change together. They had twenty-five cents to split a hamburger.

Since this was the '60s, an era of cigarette smoking as the norm, about one-half the class smoked. Some were smokers on entering school, particularly those who came from urban areas. More developed the habit during our schooling. Fortunately, some of us never did develop the smoking habit. Now, the inherent dangers of smoking are well known, and smoking is not permitted in most public places, but back then, people lit up next to you in a hospital or clinic, everywhere and anywhere. If one was allergic or did not like cigarette smoke, it was up to that person to avoid it as best they could. So accepted was smoking that MDs prescribed it for anxiety and to promote relaxation in their patients!

Cigarettes could be bought in the coffee shop from the cigarette dispenser at thirty cents a pack. A very petite nursing student was buying her pack of cigarettes when overheard was: "I didn't know they allowed twelve year olds to buy cigarettes!"

We were a cohesive group from the beginning; we had to be. Clearly, there were high expectations placed upon us. We were to set an example, since our newly formed three-year diploma school of nursing harkened back to the traditional hospital-based nursing school. But, ours was considered a "maverick" program. We were not traditional. We did not give service to the hospital in exchange for our education and room and board. So we were not "free" help like many other programs at that time. We worked for pay in the hospital, and through the three years, we advanced from nursing assistant into more of a technical nurse role. Also, how well we did would factor in for school accreditation, as the school was new and not yet accredited. The stakes were high, not just for us, but for the nursing school. The nursing school could not be accredited until it had graduated nurses who were able to pass the Minnesota State Board of Nursing examination, qualifying them to become registered nurses and receive licensure.

We paid tuition to Augsburg College for classes in the first year, and to the nursing school all three years. Of course, we also paid for our own books, uniforms, room and board, and any other expenses. While we were on the hospital unit as a student, an instructor was always with us, teaching and observing until she felt comfortable with our ability to perform procedures and care for our patients. Along with three intensive years of education, we gained "hands-on" practical knowledge working as a student, and independently, as a paid worker under the guidance of the hospital nurses.

In addition to the traditional hospital-based three-year diploma nursing school of the 1960s, there were four- and five-year bachelor of science (BSN) nursing schools. The 1970s saw another evolution in educating nurses. This was the associate degree nursing (ADN) that was part of the two-year community college program. Its focus was to educate nurses more quickly to fill the ever-present lack of nurses. The BSN or the ADN are the most typical type of program to obtain a nursing degree at this time.

We received orientation to the nursing school that was located in the westerly, walk-out basement of the hospital. There were two classrooms for lecture and a lab for hands-on learning with a hospital bed, bedding, and other medical equipment for learning nursing procedures. Miss Barber's office, as well as offices for the nursing instructors, were in this area. On the orientation tour of the hospital, we were shown the medical library, the health nurse (Miss Burry's) office, the director of nursing (Miss Lois Medima's) office, and the payroll office.

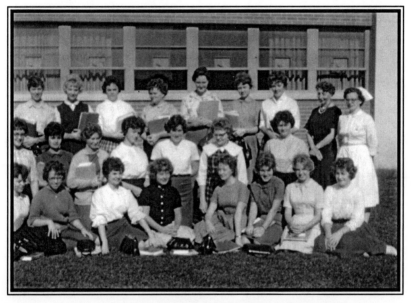

Class of 1961 outside the nursing school.
Back row: Miss Barber on (L), Mrs. Elvin on (R).

One of my most vivid memories of those first few days, so long ago, included a tour of the boiler room. I couldn't understand why we had to walk through the huge maze of pipes and valves running through the bowels of the hospital to become a nurse. It just looked like a large basement to me, but that tour ended with a big bang!

After the head boiler room man finished explaining about the pipes, etc., we went outside to the back of the hospital and stood in a grassy area. We saw a bed that held an oxygen tent, the typical way to administer patient oxygen at that time. A safety expert spoke to us on the hazards of administering oxygen and how it was a highly flammable substance. Red-colored No Smoking signs had to be posted whenever oxygen was in use on the patient room door and in the patient's room.

Then to illustrate his point, he threw a lit cigarette into the oxygen tent. I remember the loud BANG and how the tent burst into flames! A hand extinguisher was quickly used to douse the flames. So, the boiler room tour had a large impact on us all!

—Jan Kmieciak Stenson

Though we had to have had a dental exam, physical exam, and all vaccinations up to date when entering the program, another physical exam was required at the hospital. One by one, we went to Miss Burry's office, where a physician from the hospital did a brief physical exam.

Miss Burry was to give us each a mantoux (a test for TB exposure). She became very flummoxed in doing the procedure when she left the needle and syringe hanging in the arm of a student nurse while she went to answer the telephone! But, she did return from the phone call and finish the job. She was a very sweet lady, but maybe twenty-two of us were just too overwhelming. We found Miss Burry to be very open and welcoming, and we did not hesitate to visit her if we had some health issue during our tenure at Methodist. And, in our youthfulness while at the dorm, Miss Burry was affectionately referred to as "Flurry Blurry."

Within the first week of coming to Methodist, in-service education was provided for our required duties as nurse aides. After the in-service, we visited our assigned stations. It was 5A, 5B, and

4M, which were the medical units, 6A and 6B, the surgical units, special care (later called intensive care), obstetrics, labor and delivery, nursery, emergency room, orthopedics, and pediatrics.

> After listening about how to empty a urinal, make square corners, and serve trays all day long, I was relieved to get the peds assignment. When I got to the unit, the first task I was given was to feed a two-year-old child sitting in a high chair. For me, this was a piece of cake because I had a baby sister about ten years younger than me, and I'd had lots of first-hand experience with taking care of kids. It felt good to be able to do what I was asked without too much direction!
> —Jan Kmieciak Stenson

Of course, we really looked forward to our paychecks. At $1.55 per hour, we thought we really were getting a lot of money! The going rate for babysitting was fifty cents per hour.

And so, it began. We received our books and we were measured for our student uniforms. We began to learn the many acronyms in the new language of the medical world. The acronyms were very important because it wasn't long, and we were asked while working on the unit: "Go to 602, get a TPR, BP, and TCH the new surgical." This meant to go to room 602, take the temperature, pulse, respirations, blood pressure, and help the newly returned patient from surgery to turn, cough, and deep breathe.

CHAPTER 5

Augsburg College, First Semester, 1961

We began our days with devotions at 8:00 a.m. in the small first-floor hospital chapel. This was followed by religious and social aspects of nursing that was taught by Reverend Woodward, the Methodist Hospital Chaplain, on Tuesday morning. On Monday, Wednesday, and Friday, we climbed aboard the orange school bus that was waiting for us outside the front entrance of the dorm. We were off to Augsburg College to attend classes with other student nurses from Fairview, Swedish, Northwestern, Saint Barnabas, and Abbott Hospital Schools of Nursing. We returned to the dorm about 5:15 p.m. on those days. Tuesday and Thursday mornings were devoted to learning basic nursing in the hospital, and we had classroom work in the afternoons. Each day was filled with learning new concepts and a new vocabulary, sometimes with confusion, and other times with revelation!

Our Augsburg experience was memorable, as well as very demanding, and we carried a full load of challenging classes. First semester college classes included anatomy and physiology (A&P), chemistry, each with a corresponding laboratory component, and general psychology. A&P was the most attention holding and interesting, perhaps because of our professor, Dr. Mickelberg. He was a middle aged, stout, curly haired, grounded man with strong opinions, such as he would never allow his wife to work outside the home. And, if she did

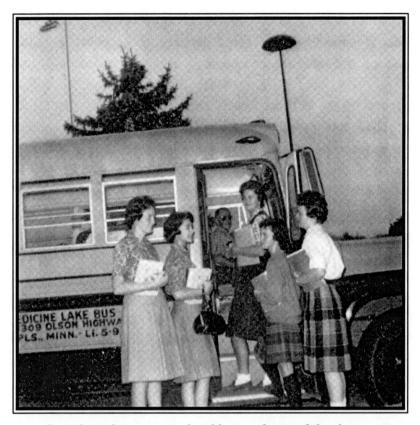

Boarding the orange school bus in front of the dorm.
(L) to (R): Beth Johnson, Sandy Johnson, Judy Mishek,
Linda Mortensbak, Velma Jean Shelton.

decide to go to work, he would quit working and stay at home! (These were probably idle threats in that era of male dominance.)

It was obvious that Dr. Mickelberg was very determined and dedicated to teaching all he could to help us in our nursing careers. He would tell us that he was there to only teach A&P, and not to include any disease processes, though it was evident that he wanted to tell us about them.

The smell of formaldehyde became very familiar in A&P lab, as well as seeing the gray-colored body organs preserved in jars. One day we had an actual human brain to touch, weigh, and examine—an incredible experience! Cell structure of the current organ being studied was covered in Dr. Mickelberg's lectures, but it seemed quite complicated, and was not easily understood. A&P required a lot of study.

The anatomy and physiology book covered every body system, beginning with the skeletal system. We began with memorizing the names of all the bones. We learned that bones have openings for major blood vessels to pass through, and that there are different shapes of bones. Flat bones compose the skull, irregular shaped bones are primarily in the spine, long bones make up the arms and legs, and short bones are in the hands and feet. Memorizing the names and locations of bones was easy. Learning the processes of how bones grow and repair themselves was a more difficult task. It became evident that physiology required critical thinking to learn the chemical and physical processes involved in the functioning of body systems.

We soon went on to the muscular system, the nervous system, followed by the circulatory, respiratory, digestive, urinary, reproductive, endocrine systems. We learned fluid, electrolyte, and acid-base balance before completing our anatomy and physiology semester.

Chemistry turned out to be quite a challenge for many of us, though we had an excellent professor, Dr. Holum. Perhaps some of us did not have as much aptitude for it, or we were not as well prepared by our high school chemistry classes. Dr. Holum had a knack for explaining and making equations seem effortless, but in spite of that fact, many of us struggled. Just like Dr. Mickelberg in anatomy and physiology, Dr. Holum wanted each of us to succeed in understanding chemistry. An interesting aspect of our chemistry class was that we sat in a large lecture hall with all the student nurses from the other hospital-based nursing programs. For those of us who struggled with chemistry, Dr. Holum provided special classes.

Our class of twenty-two had a chemistry lab, where we learned to mix different potions and record the results in a lab book. Our chemistry lab was taught by a stout Asian man who had quite a strong accent. Not only were we challenged by chemistry, but also by his speech, since we needed to get used to speech patterns that were not familiar. He wore bottle bottom glasses, and he had two gold front teeth that glistened as he told us about "easters" meaning esters, a type of carbon chain that we came to know. Vicki Lymburner Thompson recalled his explanation for how we were going to test saliva. "Spit some sawiva in te tube and taste te solution."

Wait a minute, were we supposed to taste our saliva? Then, we realized that what he was really trying to tell us was: "Test the solution (saliva) with the litmus paper!"

The general psychology class was huge and had students from the campus at large. Our professor, Dr. Anderegg, was an interesting lecturer, but she oftentimes was late in arriving to begin class. We now knew that if the professor was fifteen minutes late, we could bail out, and many times we did! And so, we became college students and we found that: "This isn't high school anymore!"

We were probably the only students on campus who were transported via an orange school bus! We learned to be on time for the bus pickup. If we weren't, it drove Mrs. Boldt and Miss Barber to anger, not a pretty scene. Eventually, we could see the streets to the campus in our sleep. While riding the bus, some of us "crammed" for exams, some slept, some played whist, and others were learning bridge from those who knew. Most of us talked or thought up pranks as the school bus rolled along. Those times on the bus helped us to learn about each other. More than once, someone would say: "We're all in this together!"

CHAPTER 6

The Uniform

Soon after our classes began, we were measured for our student nurse uniforms. One by one, we marched into the classroom for measuring. The style of the uniform had already been designed, most likely by Miss Barber and the instructors. The uniform was characteristic of nursing schools at that time, but it differed enough that it represented only our school. The uniform consisted of three parts. First, a dress was made of tiny checkered navy- and white-colored gingham cotton with large white cuffs on short sleeves and a small, white, rounded collar. Over the dress was a white skirt and a separate bib that buttoned in the back in a crisscross fashion, forming an apron over the dress. We were soon to learn that one never sat directly on the apron uniform, as it was supposed to look neat, crisp, and wrinkle-free. We were obliged to wrap the apron around in front and sit only on the dress portion.

We each had three uniforms to last the entire three years of our nursing student career. They were laundered in the hospital and starched to stand alone perfection! (A few of the students had the experience of their bibs splitting open after coming from the laundry, due to the stiff starch!) The apron had a small pocket in the front of the waistband, where we could fold our clinical assignment, keeping it handy for reference. The dress had one small breast pocket and a larger right-hand pocket just below the waistline. This pocket had a

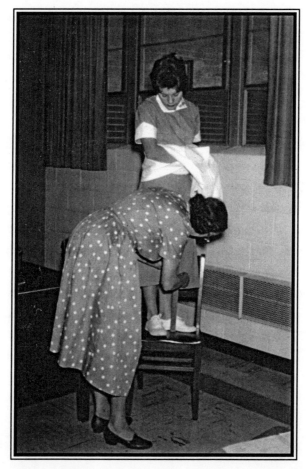

Jan Kmieciak having her student uniform measured.

flap in it, which easily held a pair of bandage scissors. We each bought our own pair of scissors for $3.50, and our instructors engraved our name on them. It felt good while carrying our scissors that we had a tool at the ready to use for cutting tape, or other tasks.

When we received our student uniforms, along with them came our name tapes. We sewed them on the upper front left side of the bib portion of our uniform so we could immediately be identified, and of course, Miss prefaced our first initial and last name. We were required to sew name tapes on the underside of the dress and skirt, mainly so they would return to the correct person from the laundry.

There were other requirements we had to meet. We could not have our hair touching the collar of our uniform, nor could we have polished fingernails. A watch with a second hand was required, but no jewelry other than a wedding or engagement ring could be worn.

Except for the nurse's cap, to which we all aspired, but had to earn, the remaining uniform code focused on white stockings and shoes. We were required to wear white hose that had seams down the back, and we were required to keep the seams straight. This, of course, was after we found some undergarment that would keep them up! At that time, there were no pantyhose. Being on our feet for eight hours of duty meant we had to wear a comfortable pair of white-laced leather oxfords.

We were proud to wear our uniform, as it gave us a feel for our chosen career. We felt identified with our profession. It wasn't until the late 1960s that pants became part of the nurses' uniform. It is rare to see a skirt uniform today. Also, today's nurse will more likely wear a "scrub" uniform. It is not unusual today for all hospital employees to be wearing scrubs differentiated by color. The patient doesn't immediately recognize who their nurse might be.

CHAPTER 7

Basic Nursing

B asic nursing incorporated medical terminology with hands-on skills. Correct spelling of medical terms was most imperative, since one letter could drastically change a meaning, such as enema and edema. The first year was the foundation year, and we learned basic information to care for patients. Our instructors told us we were being taught principles that would apply in any patient situation. One of those principles was to check the patient's vital signs (temperature, pulse, and respiration), as they were considered a "cardinal" sign, a red flag, if abnormal. Immediate medical attention could be required in that situation.

Basic nursing classes took place in the nursing school classroom. Learning to take vital signs, an important indicator of patient status, was thoroughly taught and practiced. We practiced taking temperatures with mercury thermometers. Taking an axillary temperature was totally new, while we all were familiar with oral and rectal temperatures. Finding and counting a radial pulse came fairly easily. The rate, rhythm, and strength of the pulse took on more meaning as we gained experience.

After we had learned some skills in our basic education classes, it was time to experience the first bedside patient encounter as a student nurse. We went to the medical surgical units. We listened in on report. Using the patient cardex, the off-going nurse briefed the

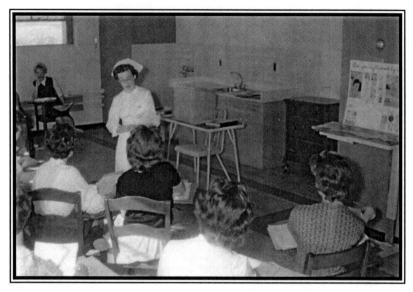

In the classroom with Mrs. Margaret Elvin.

on-coming nurses regarding each patient's care.

> I kept hearing about several patients who had had a herniorrhaphy (hernia repair.) I really didn't know what the nurse was talking about, since we'd had no surgical education yet. That would be coming in our second year. So much of this was totally foreign! However, some of the gals had worked as nursing assistants and knew the ropes better. They filled us in back at the dorm.
> —Jan Kmieciak Stenson

We learned to take a blood pressure (BP) by practicing on each other in the classroom. After a certain level of proficiency, we took the BP of a patient. We carried the portable mercury sphygmomanometer to the patient's bedside while working on the unit and listened for the BP reading with a stethoscope. The stethoscope was never carried around the neck as modern day nurses do; it was found at the nurses' station by the BP cuffs and was returned after usage. We used the stethoscope only for BPs and apical pulses. Listening for bowel or lung sounds, as well as patient teaching regarding illness, was strictly in the physician's domain.

We only had mercury measuring sphygmomanometers at that time, and self-inflating BP cuffs were way off into the future. Now, the BP equipment is mostly automatic and gives a print out not only of the patient's BP, but the pulse and respirations, as well. Technology has come to be a large part of the daily nursing routine.

Bed making was to be an art, and it was taught in the classroom. There were no fitted sheets at that time, and square corners were a must. The mattress was covered with a bed pad, and over that a sheet. At the head of the bed, we were to make a perfect square corner, and the bottom sheet was not to be tucked in at the foot. An approximately four-foot wide rubber sheet was placed horizontally across the bed, with a draw sheet of the same size placed over the rubber sheet and tucked into the sides of the mattress. The top sheet was square cornered at the foot of the bed with a thermal blanket placed on top in the same fashion. We were to check so the topside of the sheet was placed next to the patient and folded over the blanket. The hem of the sheet was not to touch the patient. We were taught how to make a bed with a patient in it and how to use the drawsheet to turn a bed patient.

Every hospital unit had a linen closet/cart. When carrying clean linens to a patient room, we were taught not to touch the clean linens to our uniform, less they become contaminated! Also, dirty linens were placed in a cloth bag, and you NEVER carried the filled bag flung over your shoulder to the dirty linen bin. But, with all the youthful exuberance, this dictate was not always followed. Unfortunately, Vera met Mrs. Terhaar, our instructor, coming around the corner one day while she was carrying the filled, dirty linen bag Santa Claus style!

Onto the bed bath. When Mrs. Elvin, our instructor, asked for a volunteer to be the patient in this classroom demonstration, one of our classmates bravely answered the call. She probably found this to be a mortifying experience to be bathed in front of her classmates. We all had much compassion for her, since any one of us could have been in her place if she hadn't volunteered. She was a good sport about the ordeal, and none of us ever forgot how to do a bed bath after that.

Nurses today rarely give a bed bath; instead, the nursing assistant will give the patient a quick once over with disposable wipes. Today's patient gets up more quickly and is in the hospital a much shorter length of time. Heart patients were on complete bed rest in the '60s. All their activities of daily living were done by the nurse, even the brushing of their teeth. The medical concept was that they should rest their heart from any extra output.

On Fridays we had a one-hour class called introduction to pharmacology. We learned about pills, tablets, capsules, and the proper way to administer them. The label of the medication (med) had to be checked three times before being administered to a patient. Giving a medication was based on the five rights:

- Right patient.
- Right time.
- Right med.
- Right dose.
- Right route of administration.

When pouring a liquid medication, you kept the bottle dosage label facing you. All of these rules helped to keep us mindful of what we were doing. We were advancing in our career when we were able to give medications to patients, and we felt good about that. With that, we also learned the huge responsibility that was involved.

After oral medications, we learned to give "shots." At first we practiced on an orange, and then on each other. There were subcutaneous injections and intramuscular injections, and they had to be administered to the correct location on the body. There were different sizes of needles and syringes, and we had to learn when to use what!

Drawing up the medication into the syringe using sterile technique had its own rules. There was much to learn and remember. Gradually we caught on, giving medications became second nature, and it was a special part of nursing care. To see easing of pain after giving a patient medication was very gratifying.

We learned a small amount of information about intravenous (IV) injection, and IV administration of medication. IV meds were rare at that time and only used in the intensive care unit (ICU). We were not taught to start IVs, and most were started by the anesthetist or an IV team of specially trained nurses.

We had heard at some nursing schools that student nurses were required to give up their chair at the nursing station if none were available to a physician. This was never requested of us at Methodist. However, there were points of decorum that we had to uphold. One of these was recognizing each other when in class or at clinical. We were not to use first names; it was always to be Miss Smith or Miss Jones.

CHAPTER 8

Working for Pay

There was no "schlukking" in H. Joan's nursing school. We came to the school on Monday, September 11th, and registered at Augsburg College on the 12th. The next day, we began classes at Augsburg and at the nursing school. On the 14th, we were introduced at the hospital banquet, bought books, and organized our lives for school and work, including readying our work uniform of a blue dress or a blue pinafore by the weekend, and studied in between. In addition to classes at Augsburg on the 15th, we went to a picnic put on by the Asbury Methodist Hospital Nurses Alumni Association. Saturday the 16th, it was a 7:00 a.m. to 3:30 p.m. orientation to work as nursing assistants, and later that week, a 3:30 p.m. to 7:00 p.m. orientation.

Miss Barber seemed to have adopted the US Army's motto of that time: "Look Sharp. Be Sharp. Go Army!" By her design, our lives were heavily structured. Rules were in place wherever they could be, and must be followed. Discipline resulted if they were not. Loyalty, duty, respect, selfless service, honor, integrity, personal courage, all US Army values, were Miss Barber's underlying values, as well.

She knew as we labored as nursing assistants, we would get to know nursing in all its many facets. We would learn and we would earn the right to become professional nurses in her school. It is also possible that her style of getting us started in nursing school, with hardly a minute to take a breath, was patterned after boot camp, minus the push-ups.

If we planned to eat and pay our tuition, working for pay was a must. Our schooling for three years cost almost four thousand dollars. The working for pay orientation included a detailed manual, and it had our schedule of work. Within this schedule of work was the statement above our names that read: "Their hours are scheduled for this semester and are not to be changed."

We were divided into three groups (A, B, and C) for continual hospital coverage. We were scheduled to work two consecutive weekends, and we had the (very looked forward to) third weekend off. One weekend we worked 7:00 a.m. to 3:30 p.m., the next was 10:00 a.m. to 7:00 p.m. The 10:00 a.m. to 7:00 p.m. shift seemed never ending; it felt like working two shifts. This was probably because we arrived in time for morning cares, then we served lunch, did afternoon tasks, served dinner, and helped with the patient bedtime routine. By the end of that shift, we had tired legs and feet, and we weren't into much Saturday night dancing, or even studying! We also worked one 3:30 p.m. to 7:00 p.m. shift during the week.

> I remember the staff nurses complaining about our odd hours and how they had to give us report about our assignment. Later, our hours were changed to coincide with the staff hours.
> —Jan Kmieciak Stenson

We had very specific duties assigned during that first year as nursing assistants. Procedures were written for each task performed, from care before meals to washing water pitchers. In the second and third years, we functioned at a nonprofessional level under the direction and supervision of a registered nurse. We were allowed to do some of the procedures for which we had been educated, and could safely accomplish, but only under very close supervision.

We did a lot of cleaning in our nurse aide role. One of our tasks was to sterilize utensils. This involved scrubbing patient wash-basins, water pitchers, and bedpans, and placing them into an auto-clave (sterilizer). Of course, we also emptied the autoclave and placed the clean utensils into the cupboard.

One day I was emptying the autoclave using a towel to lift the hot utensils, as we had been taught. All was well until I lifted a bedpan out of the rack and was raising it, when I felt a sudden excruciating pain in my right hand. Before I realized what was happen-ing, I had poured hot, boiling water over my hand! The bedpan had not been placed correctly in the au-toclave to allow the water to drain out. I wasn't re-ally sure what to do, so I continued unloading the autoclave, piled the utensils on the cart, and returned them to the cupboard.

I looked at my hand and I had huge, white, watery blisters over the tops of my fingers! I calmly walked back to the nurses' station and showed my hand to the charge nurse. She promptly sent me to the emergency room (ER), where they immediately took care of me. They poured Phixohex liquid soap over my hand. They bandaged each finger separately, and then the entire hand in soft gauze (Kerlix). I had received second-degree burns! I was worried that I wouldn't be able to work and I wouldn't have enough money for meals. Youth being on my side, I was fine in a week, soon I was back to work, and my hand had no scarring. I was concerned that I might get into trouble for this accident, but I never heard a peep from any of the "sergeants" on the unit!

—Jan Kmeiciak Stenson

While working for pay, we were able to observe the work habits and nursing styles of the floor nurses, and we gained invaluable experience doing so. Some nurses we would emulate, and others not. We had been taught many important principles of nursing that we observed were either omitted or overlooked by some of them. As an example, Jan Kmieciak Stenson stated, "I saw a staff RN put her fingers inside a convulsing patient's mouth! This was an absolute 'no-no.' She could have had her fingers bitten."

My first experience with a dying patient came when I was working as a nursing assistant on 5B during the 3:30 p.m. to 7:00 p.m. shift. A man in his early fifties had been admitted to the hospital with a leukemia diagnosis. At that time, there was very little treatment for leukemia. His body was rapidly deteriorating when I came on duty that evening. An older, seemingly deaf, RN and I were the only staff working that wing. She was not around, and she seemed to be avoiding that patient room.

I entered this man's room to introduce myself, take patient vital signs, and generally do what I could to make him comfortable. His color was very white, he had some bleeding from his nose, and he lay there motionless. I had never seen anyone appear as he did, and it was quite a shock to me, although I tried not to show it. The man's distressed wife and teenaged daughter stood at his bedside.

Feeling totally inadequate, I went to look for the nurse, but she was not to be found. A little while later, I saw the wife and daughter tearfully come out of the patient room and into the hallway. I went into the room with the wife and daughter, where this man was drawing his last breaths. He did not appear un-

comfortable as he slowly slipped away. Far more difficult for me was witnessing the raw grief of this man's family. I felt there was something we should be doing, and we had failed. With greater maturity, I realize there was little we could do but to be there.
—Carolyn Ukura Kuechle

I remember working the weekend and coming onto the unit at 10:00 a.m. I was given my typical nursing student assignment, namely, the patients no one else wanted. They figured the student nurse should have them. Of course, this also happened during the week with our clinical student nurse assignment. One morning, I had three patients needing colostomy care. This was when all colostomies had to be irrigated. Our instructor for medical rotation and myself were both up to our elbows in you know what! She decided it was a bad assignment, and I wished that she had decided that earlier.
—Judy Mishek Adams

We were very young, naïve, and unquestioning of what the "higher ups" told us. We rarely asked questions. Sometimes, with what seemed like a military approach within our nursing school, we felt we had signed on with the army! However, they did not request saluting from us. There was not a "Yes, ma'am, sergeant, major!"

Emergency Room Experiences as Related by Mary Peterson Cady
As I neared completion of my last year of high school, and was debating my career path, I decided to become a nurse for several reasons. I had considered teaching, but the cost of college was prohibitive. My mother and aunt were both registered nurses, and I had taken college prep

classes in the science and math areas. I had felt comfortable with the more difficult classes of biology, chemistry, higher algebra, and Latin with the help of my brother, and my high school advisor, Miss Stepher.

I chose to attend Methodist Hospital School of Nursing because of its location and its offer of employment. It was located only ten miles from my home. I had just graduated high school, turned eighteen, and they offered me my first job. As far as I was concerned, this was going to be a very awesome and exciting job, working as a nurse aide in the hospital emergency room! I began employment on July 5, 1961, and a future nursing school classmate, Barb, had been hired a few days earlier. We became instant friends.

I lived at home, and either my father drove me to work at the hospital or I rode the city bus that dropped me off at the bus stop on Excelsior Boulevard, directly in front of the hospital.

When I began working, I had some general orientation to the hospital and the emergency room. I found the staff very welcoming and eager to teach me all that I needed to know (a lot). Everyone at the hospital seemed very excited to have eager-to-learn nurse aides, soon-to-be nursing students, in their midst.

Located in the back of the hospital, the emergency room had its own entrance. It had a garage where a Smith Ambulance was parked and ready to leave at a moment's notice. Of course, there were several other ambulances that arrived with emergencies, and the staff was ready to care for whomever came in the door. Since there were ambulance drivers stationed at the ready, we came to know them very well. If needed, they would help us to lift patients, take a patient to the x-ray department, etc. Some of the ambulance drivers were around my age and "cute." I especially remember Mike, Josh, and "Boots," so named because he wore boots, unlike the others. There were always two trained people on each ambulance run; one was the driver, and the other was there to assist the patient.

I soon learned that the culture of the emergency room was one of teamwork and helping each other. The MDs, nurses, and nurse aides worked alongside each other, sometimes fast and furiously! There was very little hierarchy, and the comradeship was exceptional. I felt our work was very important as we helped very ill, and sometimes agitated, people, many times helping to keep them alive. I developed an awareness of the approach I needed to use with each patient: talk softly and calmly to keep that person calm, or use a much stronger voice to garner their attention.

We also had interns working and learning in the emergency room. I remember two young interns who had arrived from England. They would practice making surgical knots from outdated suture material. I learned along with them, which proved helpful later on when I was on my surgical rotation. They were a lot of fun, and we were learning "the ropes" together.

We never knew who might arrive needing care. We treated minor illnesses like rashes, sore throats, minor cuts and bruises, to heart attacks, car accidents, overdoses, and unsupervised kids getting into and swallowing medications. Unfortunately, many times, the kids shared the medication, and two and three children from the same family would have to have lavage done. This entailed having to "mummy" the child, all the while talking to him or her calmly. A large hose was inserted through the child's mouth and into the stomach to remove all contents. This was not pleasant for anyone. Sometimes the parents would stay with the child during this procedure; sometimes they would not. There were times when the child did better without the parents present.

I learned the way to the x-ray department very quickly, since I was the one to take the patients there most of the time. Sometimes, I walked them there; other times I took them by wheelchair or cart. It depended on patient condition. It was to the elevator, up to second floor, and turn left to the x-ray department. I got to know the x-ray technicians very well. We tried to guess the patient diagnosis by looking at the x-ray. Of course, we didn't say anything to the patient. That was in the MD's domain.

In the summertime, we had a lot of minor lacerations (cuts) and bruises. In winter, there were more severe car accidents and skiing accidents, usually occurring on Friday and Saturday nights. Nonetheless, it was usually busy, sometimes almost frantic! There were times the people in the waiting room became impatient, especially if they had been waiting for a long time. I couldn't blame them. But when they were told the staff was working to save the life of a heart attack victim, or that a car accident victim had just arrived by ambulance, they understood.

Some evenings when the emergency room was full of patients needing care, we worked nine to ten hours without a break. We took a bathroom break when it became absolutely necessary, but no meal breaks—no time. After we were finally done working, there were meals waiting for us in the cafeteria. The kitchen staff had put leftover meals on plates with lids over them and placed them in a warmer. We were so hungry, and they tasted so good! Forty years later, I found out that some of my high school classmates had worked in the cafeteria and had done this for us, but none of us knew about the other. I thanked them forty years later!

I worked with Ron, an orderly, who was usually very patient, kind, and helpful. One day we were cleaning instruments in hot, soapy water before autoclaving them. I asked him the name of a particular instrument. "A duckbill," he said.

Actually, it was a vaginal speculum. How wonderful to be so naïve!

We cleaned the instruments and put them in the autoclave for sterilization. Some were wrapped in a special cloth in a certain way, then fastened with a tape that had diagonal stripes. The stripes would turn blue when the instruments were totally sterilized. The date was written on the tape before autoclaving, and after one month, the sterilization became outdated. We constantly replenished equipment, IV bottles, needles, tubing, as well as ointments and medications. We also checked expiration dates on everything. The Centers for Disease

Control (CDC) and Infection Control determined expiration dates.

One time two police officers came running into the emergency room through the ambulance doors. Each officer was carrying a small child while doing mouth-to-mouth resuscitation. The children had been rescued from a fire in their foster home. The emergency room MD and several nurses worked on the children for a long time, but neither child survived.

The MD then came out of the surgical room to speak with the foster mother, who had been waiting to hear word on the children. His words to her: "Well, they're dead."

On hearing this, the foster mother fainted! I was standing next to this lady, quite a large woman, and she almost knocked me over. This physician had a rude manner and was very much wanting in his bedside skills. He helped me get this lady onto an ambulance cart to be attended.

Normally, my job as a nurse aide was to ready a body for the morgue, but one of the older nurses would not allow that. She did not want me to have memories of these children when I was so young, and might possibly have my own children. For that, I am very grateful to her.

Another time, one of the local rescue squads came driving up the long driveway from Excelsior Boulevard to the emergency room ambulance entrance. They had the siren blaring and the lights were flashing! The rescue squad was too large to fit into the ambulance garage, so they backed up to the door. They stopped, the door of the rescue squad opened, and five rescuers jumped out. They helped a mother and a little boy who had caught his mittened hand in a car door out of the vehicle. The little boy was screaming, scared, and he appeared to be in pain. One of the nurses went around the front of the desk to meet them. She very carefully removed the mitten, closely examined the child's hand, but there was no injury. After calming the child, and giving reassurance to the mother that no treatment was needed, they left the emergency room.

A little girl had shoved a hard pea up her nose. Mom and Dad couldn't get it out, so they called to say they were bringing their child into the emergency room. Again, one of the nurses met them in front of the desk. The nurse pressed her nostril and said: "Blow."

The child complied, and out came the pea!

An ambulance brought in a man who had fallen in the shower. He had cuts that needed to be sutured, and a skull x-ray was done, since he had hit his head very hard. One of the nurse aide jobs was to make out a patient clothing list. He had "no clothes," a first! I think he must have left the emergency room wearing a hospital gown with the open flap in back.

These are some of my memories of the emergency room. Much of what I learned there has been very helpful in my lifetime. What a ride! Because of this experience, I loved nursing, especially the emergency room.

—Mary Peterson Cady

CHAPTER 9

Dorm Life and Housemothers

We adapted to living together and sharing a room with another gal. We were free to decorate our rooms and move the furniture however we desired. No one had a room that looked the same as that first day when we had entered the nursing program. They were all unique and personalized.

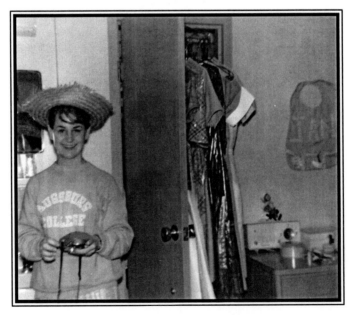

In the dorm, Monyne Jahnke.

Many students took their clothes home to be laundered. Upon returning with clean clothing in their laundry bag, some of the more ingenious students who had a liking for beer had stashed some in between their clothing! If you saw this, you kept it to yourself. Another way to bring beer into the dorm was in a hat box. The beer drinkers were very creative.

The reception desk was located at the entrance to the dorm, and there was a housemother on duty from early morning to late at night. Mrs. Boldt was the head housemother, and she lived in an apartment just down the hall. She was a widowed, thin, gray-haired, rather nervous type of woman who wore wire rim spectacles. She seemed to have great fear of Miss Barber, the nursing school director. She always wore a skirt, hose, pumps, and a prim blouse that was usually covered by a cardigan sweater.

Come to think of it, we wore much the same outfits as Mrs. Boldt. We were required to wear skirts to all classes. Pants were not a very large part of the wardrobe at that time, except for Bermuda shorts with knee-high socks and loafer shoes. Whenever a repairman had to enter second floor, Mrs. Boldt would lead the way, loudly proclaiming: "Man on Two! Man on Two!"

The housemothers were all in their late fifties or sixties, and they acted as our guards much of the time. We were required to sign out when leaving the dorm, whether for the evening, the day, or for the weekend. Also, it was very important to sign a.m. or p.m., as they kept track of such violations, which were reported to Miss Barber. There were lots of rules about when we could leave the dorm and when we had to be back. One poor student did not sign out when she went home for the weekend. Of course, this violation was reported to Miss Barber. On Monday, after the weekend, she was called to visit Miss Barber in her office and was given a two-week probation—no leaving the dorm after 7:30 p.m. for two weeks! The main dormitory door was locked at a specific time at night. Some of us got pretty clever at outsmarting the housemothers in order to get back in the dorm when we were not supposed to be out!

> Sometimes I snuck out of the dorm, after hours, by going down to the lower level of the dorm. I exited through the tunnel door that locked behind me and led into the hospital. I went to the library to study, but my focus really was to visit the "ambulance boys" whom I worked with in the emergency room. I would call my roommate when I was ready to come back to the dorm. She went downstairs and placed a piece of cardboard in the tunnel door to keep it from closing completely, and I could get back into the dorm without having to walk past the housemother. She never suspected. I suppose I looked too innocent to be guilty of any such behavior!
> —Mary Peterson Cady

Another situation involving housemothers was when Velma decided to use the dorm window in the lounge area on second floor to dry her starched nursing cap.

> The evening before the Joint Commission of Accreditation for Healthcare (JCAH) was to be visiting at the hospital, I decided to wash and starch my nursing cap. Instead of attaching my starched cap to the glass provided for drying, I decided it would be more convenient to dry it on the lounge window of the dorm. I placed it low in the corner of the window, where I was sure it couldn't be seen from Excelsior Boulevard. I was wrong about it not being seen. Mrs. Boldt, our housemother, became quite upset after she saw it. She called all of us together on the lower level of the dorm and wanted to know who

was responsible for doing such a thing when we all were well aware of the JCAH visit! None of my fellow classmates betrayed me, even though they knew I had done it. Mrs. Boldt threatened to ground all of us, unless someone admitted it. I confessed and spent the next few weeks grounded and signing in every evening.

—Velma Jean Shelton

By the time we were in our third year, there were often long goodbyes between lovers in the entryway. What did the housemothers think of that, since they had a clear view from the reception desk! Perhaps it brought them back to their youth. Maybe the many rules they produced for us were to keep us tuned into the respectable avenue of nursing in all facets of our lives.

A buzzer system sounded in the dorm when a student had a phone call or a visitor. There was a different buzz for each. If both phones in the hallway were busy, one was obliged to go down to the housemother's desk to talk on the phone. This was something none of us wanted to do! If we had a call, and didn't come to the phone, we were paged by the housemother. In the evenings, a plump, gray-haired, grandma-like lady with a slurred speech pattern sat at the reception desk. When she used the intercom to page, it was quite difficult to determine what she was saying, as it all ran together. "Vahlakamp" was one particular pronunciation that we heard (for student Vera Kemp)!

Someone was always studying and sometimes it just got to you! Some of us played pranks, like quietly pouring water under a "too much studying" person's door until it was noticed, or we sang loudly in the hallway until we got their attention! Really, it was time to have some fun already!

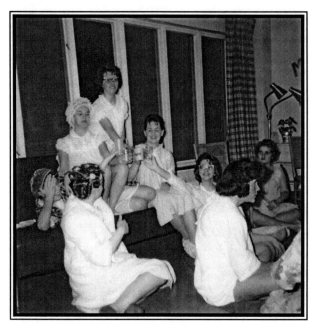

Dorm life. Just hanging out.

One day, needing to "let loose" during finals, Betty Beard and Vera Kemp took the laundry cart from third floor and brought it to second floor via the elevator. Betty got in the cart and Vera covered her with clothing. Vera ran the cart up and down the dorm hallway several times, and then Betty popped up from underneath the clothing! Suddenly, Mrs. Boldt appeared out of nowhere! She had a very "stern look" on her face. They were instructed by Mrs. Boldt to return the cart to where they had found it. Mrs. Boldt later admitted that this incident was very funny, and she had struggled to keep a straight face, let alone a stern one.

Some of us studied in any quiet area we could find to get away from the second floor dorm chaos. We went to the hospital boardrooms or the hospital library. The problem with that was that you had to be dressed to go there, and if you had already gotten into lounge type clothing, you would have to throw your coat over you. Of course, if you wanted to get a snack from the coffee shop, it was the same deal.

(No wonder we liked having some snacks in the windows.)

We discovered third floor was a good place to study in a quieter atmosphere, and we didn't have to be properly dressed or wear a coat! Not all of third floor was finished at the time, and it had a practice lab. Mrs. Chase, the mannequin used for positioning and bathing, lay on the hospital bed. On occasion, she was used for a prank. One evening she was dressed in pajamas, including hair rollers and cap (our usual bedtime attire) over her hair. She was placed in Vera Kemp's bed, properly positioned for sleeping with the bed covers up to her neck, while Vera was in the library studying. When Vera returned from studying and walked into her room, she was perplexed when she saw who she thought must be her roommate in her bed. We were elated to see the joke had worked when she said: "What is Betty doing in my bed?"

The skeleton, "Elmer," also lived in that room on third floor. We learned about bones and bone markings by studying him.

Two out-of-town gals had cars parked in the parking lot in front of the dorm. Beth Johnson from Wisconsin had her own car, and Karen Miller from southern Minnesota drove a 1953 Chevy. Their cars came in very handy for some of the rest of us for grocery runs, going to the movies, a late-night drive to McDonald's, or other nearby places. Of course, the late night drive to McDonald's involved sneaking in and out the tunnel door. We appreciated being invited and being part of the mobility their cars allowed.

> One very cold, winter night when we got
> out to the parking lot for a McDonald's run, there sat
> Beth's car with a very flat tire. Changing that tire with
> the cold wind blowing is a memory I won't forget!
> —Judy Mishek Adams

Across Excelsior Boulevard south of Methodist Hospital was the beautiful Meadow Brook Golf Course. It had a perfect sliding hill that was almost directly across from the dorm. We took cafeteria food trays and paper boxes to use for sleds, and off we went on the short walk through the parking lot across Excelsior Boulevard, into the golf course, and up the hill. It was an exhilarating way to spend a winter evening as we joyfully slid down that hill!

There were bikes at the dorm that we could sign out and ride. They were handy for grocery shopping for those of us who did our own cooking at the dorm. Betty Beard remembers riding from the grocery store with a bag of apples hanging on the handlebar. They fell off the bike, and they rolled all over busy Excelsior Boulevard! So ended that bag of apples.

Dr. and Mrs. Hoffert were very kind to us in every way. Dr. Hoffert was very patient with student nurses during surgery. He never yelled or belittled our efforts when we were scrubbed in with him. Mrs. Hoffert was paramount in helping in the flower garden behind the dorm, and she encouraged us to be involved in the garden club. They invited us to their home for lovely dinners. At the time, we probably didn't realize what a large undertaking all that they did for us had to be for them.

Methodist Hospital and associates were all very welcoming to a group of twenty-two young women in the first class of the new nursing program. The Methodist ministers invited us to a dinner in the hospital cafeteria where we were individually introduced. The Asbury nurse Alumni Association had a picnic for us at the home of Mrs. Swanson. Methodist Hospital Chaplain Reverend Donald Woodward and Mrs. Woodward invited us to their home at Christmastime for a party with food, singing, and making corsages.

CHAPTER 10

The Pink Ladies

The Pink Ladies were a very important part of our life at Methodist. Most were probably in their fifties and sixties, and they were volunteers who lived in the community. Of course, they always wore pink while on duty at the hospital. They helped out in all areas of the hospital, from working in the coffee and gift shop, taking care of the information desk, running errands, visiting patients, and generally doing whatever was asked of them. They smiled, looked pretty in pink, and seemed to enjoy life! When studying, working, and having all the stresses of becoming a nurse piled up, we looked at them and said: "I want to be a Pink Lady!"

Shortly after our arrival at Methodist, we were invited to an introduction tea with the Pink Ladies. At the tea, we met our assigned Pink Lady, who was to become our "Big Sister." Miss Barber, no doubt, had a lot of input into which Pink Lady would be assigned to which student. The Pink Ladies "adopted" us, and they invited us to their homes for wonderful homemade dinners with their families. They took us out to dinner, and to the movies, and were very supportive and kind. They had even set up a fund in the nursing school where they loaned money on a short-term basis if we were short in paying tuition, or for other emergency needs. The Big Sister concept was prevalent in nursing schools at the time. There were no students before us, since we were the first class. We became Big Sisters to the second class, who came into the nursing school a year later.

Teas were new to most of us, and for the most part, we had not been acculturated to them. They were, as they sound, a bit stuffy, and a part of Miss Barber's focus in trying to make us well-rounded individuals. She wanted to allow the opportunity for "social intercourse" as taught in her class. At the tea, there were little bites of food to eat, along with coffee or tea to drink. We were to sip our tea or coffee, have a little bite of food to eat, and very properly visit with all who had gathered.

> At the Big Sister introduction tea, I wasn't accustomed to drinking coffee or tea. I opted for coffee, loaded it with sugar and cream, and had all I could do to drink it. After that, I learned to drink black coffee!
> —Judy Mishek Adams

Mrs. Hamilton was a Pink Lady who became our choir director. She had a music background, and had been a choir director. She was very light hearted and fun, and we enjoyed her! We practiced weekly in the ground floor recreation room, all twenty-two of us. We sang a wide variety of music, but there was a song that went, "I'm a girl and by me that's only great / I am glad that my silhouette is curvy." When there was an objection to singing this song by probably the curviest nursing student, Mrs. Hamilton listened. We no longer sang this song. This, most likely, was another reason we enjoyed her so much. She was quite refreshing as she listened to us, and she didn't just dictate.

During the Christmas season, we had several singing engagements. We sang for the Board of Governor's dinner, the employee party in the cafeteria, the physician's dinner party, Asbury Methodist for the geriatric residents, and we caroled in the hospital hallways for two hours one night.

During this time, playing a bongo drum was a common fad among college-age students. I just happened to have brought my brother's set of bongo drums from home after our Thanksgiving break. The drums were small, and I sat holding them between my knees to play. Well, one of the songs we sang for the physician's dinner party was, "The Little Drummer Boy." I had a part to learn on the drums for that song. It all went well, and I was lucky to be hidden behind my standing classmates as I beat the drums!

—Jan Kmieciak Stenson

CHAPTER 11

Second Semester, January 1962

All twenty-two of us made it into the second semester of nursing school that January of '62, some of us by the skin of our teeth! In this second semester, we had four college classes at Augsburg College, and we rode the orange school bus four days a week. Our classes at Augsburg were microbiology, nutrition, communications, and sociology. Microbiology was the one difficult science class that would require our utmost attention, in comparison to the other three classes. Microbiology had a separate lab component, as well.

When we returned from Augsburg each day, we had a basic nursing class lecture. Combined with the four college classes, plus the classes and clinical at Methodist, we had a very heavy schedule. We worked for pay in the hospital one evening a week, and two out of three weekends.

Our classes at Augsburg began January 31; however, on January 29, half of the class was summoned to Miss Barber's office. We were given the news that we were on probation until we got our grade point up and that, of course, meant until the end of the semester when grades were given. This meant we must study from 5:00 p.m. to 9:00 p.m. every weekday night, and we had to be in by 10:30 p.m. on the weekends. It was high-rolling stress and lots of pressure! None of us could afford to get another D!

Microbiology was taught by Dr. Nash, and just as Dr. Mickelberg and Dr. Holum, he knew his subject backward and forward, and he, too, really cared that we firmly grasped the subject. He had a gentle way of explaining topics to make them not only interesting, but easy to comprehend. We took the class with other freshmen nursing students from the surrounding hospitals. There must have been two hundred or more students in "Old Main" watching and listening to Dr. Nash as he explained different organisms and how they caused disease. It was a fascinating subject.

During our microbiology lab, we learned to use the microscope to identify bacteria, yeast, fungus, and other types of cells. At first, it was difficult to see anything under the microscope, but as we practiced, it all came into focus. Our lab final project was to identify an organism. This meant that we had to run numerous lab tests to recognize the microbe. By the end of class in May, we had all finished satisfactorily.

Our nutrition class was taught by a tall, plain, and lean woman with huge feet. She wore large, brown, laced-up oxford shoes. She had a very curious way of pronouncing protein. It sounded as if she was saying, "pro-dee-end." In our first assignment, we were to keep track of everything we ate for a week. We had to graph every component of the food on a huge chart, breaking down the calories, minerals, vitamins, etc.

I was one not to eat breakfast so I could stay in bed a little longer. One day I had a cherry Life Saver for breakfast, peanut butter on an apple for lunch, and chicken hot dish for dinner. Most of these foods were easy to graph into their food components, except the chicken hot dish with its many ingredients. Nutrition was interesting, and we learned how to

practice better nutrition. It helped to lay a foundation that we could use in teaching patients about how
nutrition influenced health.
—Jan Kmieciak Stenson

Our communications class found us having to create and give
speeches, write papers, write letters in correct form, read books, and
give reports. In that class alone, there was plenty to occupy our time.

It seemed by the time we got to study sociology, there was
little time left. It became a "cram" class: cram in as much as you can to
pass the test, and move on.

CHAPTER 12

The Capping Ceremony

When we had received our student nurse uniforms on October 21, 1961, we had also received three caps that were in the same design as the Asbury Methodist nursing school. They would complete our nursing uniform, but they would not be worn until after our capping ceremony. After laundering the caps, we placed them in heavy starch and put them to dry on the old storm window in the second floor lounge. Mrs. Elvin, one of our instructors, was an Asbury Methodist grad, and she showed us how to properly fold our caps.

In the mid-1800s, Florence Nightingale, a nurse during the European Crimean War, saw the importance of nursing as she volunteered to care for the wounded soldiers. Though the profession of nursing had been around for centuries, she recognized the need to bring professionalism to it. Miss Nightingale was instrumental in requiring that nurses be welled trained, and she defined the need of a uniform to give the nurse a professional look.

The nursing cap became part of the uniform, and it evolved from the veil of the nun's habit to give tribute to the many nurse nuns, the earliest nurses. Women of the earlier times usually had long hair, and it required a veil or wrap to keep their hair out of the way while doing nursing tasks. The cap was instituted to keep the nurse's hair neatly in place, and to present a modest appearance. It became a symbol of one of the noblest professions, and also signifies dignity, dedication, and educational attainment.

The milestone event for which we had long been hoping, not just this school year, but in earlier years when we had dreamed of becoming nurses, occurred on Friday, February 23, 1962, at 8:00 p.m. We were thrilled to be at our capping ceremony at Aldersgate Methodist Church, several blocks east of the hospital in Saint Louis Park! Our parents, family, friends, some hospital staff, and faculty were seated in the pews to watch. One by one, each of us went up to the altar to receive the nursing cap from Mrs. Margaret Elvin, nursing instructor. We sang "You'll Never Walk Alone," "I Believe," and "Perfect Prayer." Miss Carola Haaland, nursing instructor, led us in the recitation of the Florence Nightingale Pledge.

Miss H. Joan Barber, the director of the school of nursing gave the following address:

Class of 1964: Tonight you have received your caps. They are the symbol of your profession, the identification of your school, and you have pledged yourselves to practice your profession faithfully.

It will be well for you to think carefully of the words which you have spoken, for they carry with them a great responsibility. With effort, and some small sacrifices on your part, you have now achieved the first step toward becoming professional nurses. As you go on your way, it will be increasingly necessary for you to remember that you are here, primarily, not to get what you can for yourselves, but to try to make the lives of others happier and easier.

In the long run, your attitudes will give depth and direction to your behavior, and will communicate more about you, and how you feel toward others, than your words do. For it is true that the more you forget yourselves in the service of others, the greater will be your own satisfactions and rewards.

And there lies the dividing line between the "worker" and the truly professional person. It is the difference between just working and serving, that ability to give greatly of yourselves in the service of others.

As members of the first class of Methodist Hospital School of Nursing, you have a unique opportunity.

If you set your standard of service high, and keep it there, and still maintain the compassion and eagerness which you already possess, you can be an inspiration and help to the classes which follow. In truth, that is one of your most serious responsibilities.

You will have a great many conditions to meet, and adjustments to make; there is no doubt about that. But you have a great store of knowledge from those who have gone before you. If you keep an open mind, an inquiring mind, your way will be pleasant and profitable, not a penance, but a delight.

So few people succeed greatly, because so few people can conceive a great end and work toward that end without deviating and without tiring. We all know the man who works day and night for money, and gets rich, and the man who works day and night for whatever goal he sets for himself, and reaches that goal.

So, on this evening of your dedication, each of you must evaluate clearly what her own particular goal is, and then determine to work toward that goal without deviating and without tiring.

If you can, and will, do that one thing, you will be welcome members not only of Methodist Hospital School of Nursing, but of the entire nursing profession, as well. So wear your cap proudly and with dignity, remembering always that it is a symbol of your service to humanity.

—H. Joan Barber, Director, School of Nursing

THE FLORENCE NIGHTINGALE PLEDGE

I solemnly pledge myself before God and in the presence of this
    assembly
to pass my life in purity and to practice my profession faithfully.
I will abstain from whatever is deleterious and mischievous
and will not take or knowingly administer any harmful drug.
I will do all in my power to maintain and elevate the standard of
    my profession
and will hold in confidence all personal matters committed to my
    keeping
and family affairs coming to my knowledge in the practice of my
    calling.
With loyalty will I endeavor to aid the physician in his work,
and devote myself to the welfare of those committed to my care.

Written by: Lystra Gretter, Nursing Instructor
Detroit, Michigan, 1893

Today this pledge, or a variation of it, continues to be used in some nursing school settings at graduation or pinning. There no longer is a capping ceremony, as caps have become outmoded. The reasons for this are the hazards of infection control and use of technological equipment, caps being cumbersome, and today there are many male nurses in the profession who would not wear caps.

In my day, I relished wearing my cap, and it gave me something to attain. I always felt more complete with my cap perched on my head, as it said to all, "I'm a real nurse."
—Jan Kmieciak Stenson

Now we surely at least looked like nurses! And, it was back to work studying and "cramming" for more tests.

Next year, our class would cap the new freshmen class, as we would be "Big Sisters" to them. Paired with a new student, we had the opportunity to guide them through what it was like to be a nursing student.

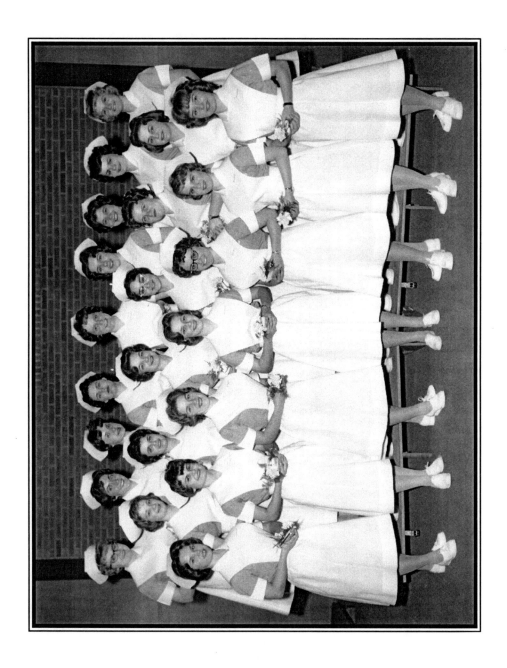

Singing at Hennepin Avenue Methodist Church.
Back row (L) to (R): Judy Stoneback, Judy March, Betty Beard,
Judy Mishek, Beth Johnson, Karen Velte, Vera Kemp,
Velma Jean Shelton, and Irma Lobnitz. Middle row:
Carolyn Ukura, Barbara Carlson, Vicki Lymburner,
Sandra Johnson, Barbara Wyland, and Monyne Jahnke.
Front row: Linda Mortensbak, Sue Tingerthal, Jan Kmieciak,
Mary Peterson, Karen Young, Sue Lehmeyer, and Sandra Morrow.

CHAPTER 13

Basic Nursing II

In basic nursing II, we began to do more nursing procedures during clinical. We gave injections, inserted Foley urinary catheters, changed dressings, and of course, gave bed baths.

As we gained experience, we were being looked on as being more valuable to the nursing team during our scheduled work for pay shifts. They welcomed us when we arrived on the unit, and depended on us, knowing that we could well perform tasks given to us. During the evening shift, one of our first duties was to give back rubs. It was up one side the hall and down the other, and every patient received a back rub. This was also a good time to introduce ourselves and get to know the patients.

Sue Tingerthal began working at downtown Asbury Methodist with the geriatric patients during the second semester. Her home was nearby, and she could ride the bus from her home during the three-month summer break. Sue found this experience to be quite interesting and enjoyable, and she encountered the humor found in the nursing home situation. One day, a little lady lying in bed with a restraint jacket to prevent her from falling, quite loudly said: "One thing the doctor ordered is that I should breathe!"

In the current long-term care facility, a jacket restraint is no longer used.

During that spring of 1962, we were finishing up our coursework at Augsburg College. A whole lot hinged on how well we did with our final testing there, even whether a second year of nursing school would be forthcoming.

> It was in the middle of spring finals for Augsburg College when everyone was getting crazy with all the studying we had been doing. Someone got the idea to take a break and go to Lake Calhoun. There was no car available, so we decided to call a cab. I don't remember how many of us squeezed into the cab, but it was pretty crowded. We piled in layers so we all could get in. We split the cab fare, each of us paying approximately thirteen cents each way, a very good deal, we thought! When the cab driver dropped us back at the dorm, he told us not to call the company in the future. They would not take so many of us in one cab again.
> —Velma Jean Shelton

At the end of second semester, we had completed a total of 395 clock hours of college classes and 148 hours of nursing classes. We were on our way!

CHAPTER 14

Summer Break, June 1962

By Jan Kmieciak Stenson

We had finally finished our first year of nursing school! Phew! We all were in need of rest and relaxation (R&R). Mrs. Hamilton, our choir director, kindly invited us to her cabin "up north" near Crosby, Minnesota, for a weekend of fun. Most of our class accepted the invitation, and we piled into three cars and headed for the lake. We took along bathing suits, thongs (better known today as flip-flops), tanning lotion (sunscreen was not in style), shorts, tube tops, and of course, cigarettes for those of us who smoked.

Having grown up in Chicago, I had never been to the north country of Minnesota. Watching the tall, beautiful trees and the blue, sparkling lakes as we drove north from the Twin Cities was quite an exciting sight for me! Vera Kemp was driving the car that I was riding in, and there were six of us in it. We stopped at a park near Lake Mille Lac where there was a huge replica of a fish. Next, we stopped at a drive-in where there were many kinds of homemade pies. I chose lemon meringue, my favorite. It was the most delicious pie that I have ever eaten! And, the price wasn't bad either, at only seventy-five cents for a piece of pie. Just the excitement of getting away, and no studying, probably enhanced all that we were experiencing.

We piled back into the cars and rode for another hour. We listened to the radio and sang along to songs like "Big Girls Don't Cry" and "Duke of Earl." Then we turned down a long gravel road that led to the Hamilton cabin. A large, beautiful cabin came into view near a glistening lake. The cabin was equipped with a large kitchen, full laundry, living room, and bedrooms. There also was a bunk house with bunks stacked three high, and that's where I slept. That night when we turned in, I remember hearing the humming of mosquitoes outside. It sounded like a huge herd of mosquitoes right outside my window.

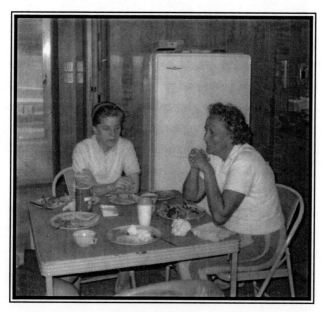

Jan Kmieciak and Mrs. Hamilton at kitchen table.
Hamilton Cabin, Crosby, Minnesota.

Mrs. Hamilton provided the food for us all. Her son and one of his friends were there to help with the boats, fishing, and the muscle work. We spent the next day outside swimming, boating, canoeing, working on tans, and riding the jeep through the woods. The guys were adept at handling the sailboat, "The Sunfish," and many of us got our first experience in sailing. "Prepare to come about," was the first command we learned, and this was to turn the sailboat. The weather was perfect, lots of sun, eighty-five degrees, and just the right amount of breeze to sail along leisurely! Most of us wanted to be outside to get that coveted Coppertone tan.

Judy March, a beloved classmate, was experienced at water skiing. She made it a priority that all who wanted would get up on skis. She stood in the water up to her waist near the dock and helped each novice to get the skis on just right. Judy was determined to see us ski, and she didn't give up. She knew just how to get the towrope situated, and how to position us for success. "Hit it!"

She yelled to the driver of the boat when the skier was positioned just right. The boat zoomed off, and sometimes I got up, and sometimes not. Usually, it took more than one try to get up on the skis. When I thought I was sure to get up, down I'd find myself, into the clear blue deep. I remember the first time I was up and gliding over the water. It was an exhilarating feeling of skiing in that crouched position that Judy made sure I could do. How long could I stay up? "Yikes! I can't hold on anymore. Will I drown, or just get water up my nose?"

We didn't have life vests, just a foam rubber belt around the waist that worked pretty well to help stay afloat when, inevitably, we fell into the deep. We were so proud to say, at the end of the day, that we could water ski!

Sadly, Judy left us all too soon. She was in her early forties when she became ill with lung cancer. It took her much too quickly, and she left her husband and two young sons without her wonderful, joyous smile and the great knack of seeing the best in everyone.

The Hamilton cabin was located in a forested area, where it was incredibly beautiful with the trees, sky blue water, and purple-gold sunsets. We spent the nights eating, talking, playing cards, and of course, putting Noxzema on our sunburned bodies. A new card game that we played was called "spoons," since when receiving two or three of a kind, we grabbed spoons.

There was no TV to watch at the cabin. We cranked up the radio and most of us danced. It was the "Bristol Stomp" and the very popular at the time "Twist" to the music of Chubby Checkers and

Fats Domino. Another song, "Sherry," really made us feel like dancing, in spite of being tired after all the physical activity of the day. The "stroll" was a dance that was seen on the TV show, *American Bandstand*. It was popular in the east, but we rarely danced it.

We wanted it to go on forever!

When it was time to leave that Sunday, we all felt refreshed, but sore from using muscles we didn't know we had and aching from sunburn. But, oh well, we'd soon have a great tan. After all, being tanned as dark as possible was really "in style." We'd had the perfect end to that first memorable year together as we had learned our profession. Now, we looked forward to "no studying," and earning money to spend, and to save, for the next school year.

Apparently, Mrs. Hamilton hadn't approved this cabin weekend with Miss Barber. Unfortunately, when Miss Barber found out about it, Mrs. Hamilton was no longer our choir director.

PART TWO

THE SECOND YEAR, SEPTEMBER 1962

CHAPTER 15

Surgery Rotation

By: Jan Kmieciak Stenson

"Believe you can, and you're halfway there."
—Theodore Roosevelt

We were feeling comfortable, and much more confident, beginning our second year of nursing school. The first few weeks starting the program the previous year, we had felt excitement, a bit of fear, some anxiety, and trepidation as we had begun our path into the unknown.

Our summer had been spent working, saving money, and gaining patient experience. In the second year, we were considered juniors, and a new class of forty-four freshman entered the school. We were excited to be the "wise ones" as we welcomed them to the school. They lived on the dormitory floor above us, which meant we no longer could escape to third floor! We became their "Big Sisters," continued the scavenger hunt tradition from the Hamline-Asbury Methodist nurses, and entertained them periodically during their first year.

A complete surgical suite was located on second floor of the hospital. It was comprised of six operating rooms, a cast room, two cystoscopic rooms, and a post-anesthetic recovery room (PAR) for twenty patients. The x-ray department, laboratory, central supply, and pharmacy were also located on second floor.

In this year, we would be doing our six-week surgery rotation, eleven students at a time. We actually would be scrubbed in and helping in patient operations! This was a very exciting thought for some of us, and a most "scary" thought for others.

Even writing about this surgery rotation almost fifty years later gave me the "willies." Remembering back to that time, I'd had scary thoughts such as: What if I should hand the surgeon the wrong instrument, he doesn't notice, and damage is done to the patient? I'm not sure if I can handle seeing that much blood. I might faint, possibly fall into the surgical site, and contaminate everything. The surgery will stop, and they will have to haul me out of there. Maybe I will screw up on sterile technique, the surgeon will yell at me, and I will have caused the patient an infection. I am totally afraid of the scary surgeon stories. Can some surgeons really be that way? I don't want to find out.

So, maybe I can just opt out of this rotation. And that, of course, was not just a wild thought, but a totally wild fantasy.

Resigned to my fate, I checked the surgery schedule the night before. If I was to be with one of the scary surgeons, I hardly slept all night. In the morning, I ate very little breakfast in the event that I might vomit, and I arrived on time at the surgery suite to don scrubs and scrubbed in. I felt very lucky if I was going to be in the operating room with one of the favored surgeons, and hoped not to get the one who yelled, "Rankin" (a surgical instrument), who if given the wrong instrument, would just throw it. It's hard to remember if he threw it at the nurse, or just at the nearest wall.

—Carolyn Ukura Kuechle

One of the first things we learned is that we had to wear conductive shoes that had special soles to decrease static electricity while we were working in the surgical area, since many of the anesthetics used in surgery were flammable. Another requirement was that we had to wear cotton slips underneath our uniforms, rather than nylon, to reduce static electricity, as well. Slips, what are those? We might ask in today's world.

We had to wear our entire student nurse uniform to the surgical area and then change into scrub dresses. The surgical area was quite cold, temperature-wise, and the scrub dresses were not very warm. Everyone had their hair covered at all times, with usually a white cotton head "adornment." Of course, we all had to wear a white mask that covered our nose and mouth. With the mask on our face, it was difficult to identify a student or staff member. One nursing school instructor circulated through the many operating rooms, but staff members took us under their wings to show us what we needed to learn and do during this experience. We were never allowed to be the only scrub nurse. There was always a staff member working with us, and that gave us a certain sense of security.

I loved being in surgery because I felt like I was really doing something useful. The scrub nurse was usually a licensed practical nurse (LPN) or a scrub tech. Their job was to hand instruments to the surgeon as he performed the surgical procedure. The RN's role was to circulate in the operating room. She was responsible for documenting the sponge count, patient blood loss, and numerous other tasks during the procedure.

We had heard "horror" stories of how surgeons would sometimes throw instruments, yell at staff, or tell "dirty" stories

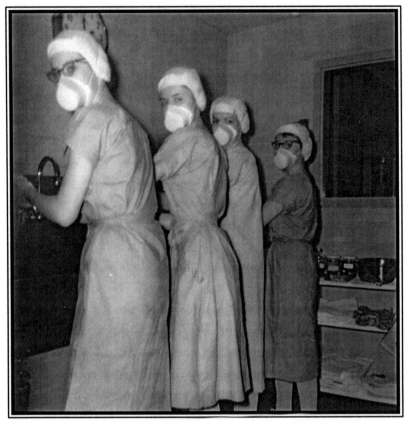

Ten-minute scrub before working in surgery.

during surgery. We were all on guard.

I was watching a thyroidectomy (removal of the thyroid gland) when the surgeon pointed to the trachea and asked me what was the name of that structure. I gulped out the correct word, and then he promptly forgot that I was there.

Everything done in the operating room was oriented toward preventing infection in the patient. It was where we learned very strict sterile technique. The scrub nurse was responsible for all sterile equipment, while the circulating nurse took charge of all nonsterile items. If there was any possibility that a sterile item was contaminated, it was discarded immediately. No questions asked!

Before entering the operating room, we learned to do a ten-minute scrub. It began with cleaning the fingernails, then using a brush to scrub the nails, the palms, back of hands, around the wrists, and up the arms to above the elbows. This was the initial scrub of the day. If you went to another operating room for another case, you only had to do a five-minute scrub. Remembering that you never scrubbed up and down your arms to prevent contamination, I saw many doctors scrub this way. I was amazed!

After scrubbing in, we learned how to put on our sterile gown and gloves. We did the closed gloving technique by actually opening the sterile gown package and then getting the gloves on our hands by manipulating the sleeves of the gown. This took practice!

We also learned to "glove" the doctors and help them on with their surgical gown. Gloving was a real trick to do and took lots of practice to do it effectively. Some of the students brought gowns and gloves back to the dorm to practice.

Not only did the operating room staff scrub for surgery, but the patient was scrubbed! And, I mean scrubbed vigorously! Wherever the operative site might be, the circulating nurse performed a ten-minute scrub. Beginning with the operative site and moving outward, round and round the circulating nurse scrubbed while using a special tray of equipment. Most of the scrub time was spent on the operative site and less on the surrounding area. If an appendectomy (removal of appendix) was being performed, the scrub area started at the nipple line and went on to the mid-thigh region.

Another important task was learning to position and drape a patient for surgery. Many sterile sheets were used to maintain a sterile field, and specific sterile principles were used. Some of these principles were: the edge of anything is not sterile; only sterile items can touch sterile items; anything wet is not sterile.

The operating rooms contained lots of equipment, gas machines, scales, buckets, hundreds of various tubes, and all manner of instruments. We were to identify and learn the purpose of all the equipment. Probably the first we learned to identify was the kelly, a hemostat for "bleeders." There was the curved kelly, the Kutner, and the Metzenbaum.

When handing a knife (scalpel) to the surgeon, it was held with blade down, handle toward the surgeon's hand so as not to cut him. Once an instrument was used on the skin, it was not reused inside the patient's body, since organisms from the skin could be transmitted internally. We got to know retractors very well because we usually were holding or pulling on them so the surgeon could see into the surgical site. Holding the Balfore retractor became the student nurse's main role. We arranged all instruments and lined them up in the order of use on the Mayo stand. Working in the operating room helped us to learn organizational skills and to appreciate how surgical procedures could help the patient.

A very important task during surgery is keeping track of the sponge count! It was necessary to count every item used in an operation before and after the procedure to verify that no items are left within a patient. Things got fairly bloody in some surgeries, and a four-by-four sponge could easily be saturated and go unnoticed. It was our job to help make sure that didn't happen.

I remember helping with a mastectomy (breast removal), and I watched as the surgeon got deeper into the area. I thought he had forgotten a sponge, and I knew I had to tell him. But did I, a lowly student, have the courage to speak up? Finally, I told him, lest the sponge count be wrong. To my surprise, the surgeon was very grateful for the interruption. After that, Dr. Maxeiner and I got along just great.

Suture was another curious item. Some were absorbable and others were not, hence needing removal after several days. They came in small packages with numbers (2/0 chromic, 5/0 cardiac.) The needles were atraumatic and had either a cutting edge or soft edge. The cutting edge needles were used primarily on the skin, and the soft edge needles were used on soft tissue like the intestine. There were wire sutures used in orthopedic conditions.

There were many differences fifty years ago compared to today's medical and surgical world. Surgical patients came into the hospital the night before surgery and often stayed five days or more, depending on the surgical procedure.

There were no instruments for doing any kind of endoscopic procedures. All patients in need of a cholecystectomy (removal of gall bladder) had about a ten-inch incision that was made along the right rib cage to expose the gall bladder region underneath the liver. Often these patients had a T-tube to drain bile in place, as well as a large dressing over the operative site upon return from surgery. These patients had great difficulty coughing and deep breathing after surgery. Our instructors drilled into us the importance of TCH (turn, cough, and hyperventilate) the post-op patient.

Some of us were lucky to see cataract removal. The preparation for this surgery was incredible by today's standards. First, the eyebrow was shaved, then the eyelashes clipped, and in surgery, the circulating nurse scrubbed the eye area very thoroughly with surgical soap. After surgery, the patient had to lie still and could not move her/his head in any direction. Sandbags were placed on either side of the patient's head to prevent movement.

Sue Tingerthal had just begun her surgery rotation when one weekend when the dorm phone rang shortly after midnight. There had been a car accident and help was needed in surgery. She donned her uniform and went straight to the operating room area, where she got into scrubs. A patient's arm had a severed tendon. Sue scrubbed in, and ended up holding the patient's arm in one position for about two hours straight! Finally, another nurse came to relieve her. Very soon after that, Sue was back in her bed where, exhausted, she slept for many hours.

During our surgery rotation, we learned about the human body inside and out. This was invaluable knowledge when taking care of patients after surgery. No wonder they had pain. Now, we had more tools to care for our patients.

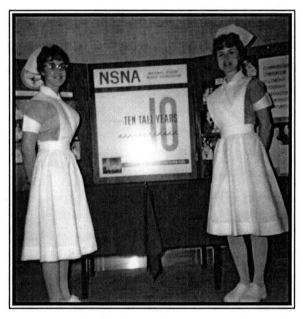

Taking leave of it all, Sandy Johnson and Betty Beard
are off to Atlantic City, New Jersey, as our delegates to the
National Student Nurse Association.

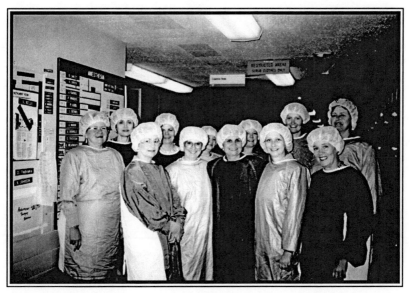

At the entrance to the surgical suite, twenty-five-year
reunion tour. (L) to (R): Barb Wyland, Betty Beard,
Monyne Jahnke, Velma Jean Shelton, Sue Lehmeyer,
Carolyn Ukura, Sue Tingerthal, Vicki Lymburner,
Mary Peterson, Beth Johnson, Jan Kmieciak, and Judy Mishek.

CHAPTER 16

Medical and Surgical Rotation (Med/Surg)

By: Jan Kmieciak Stenson

Besides our surgery rotation, the largest part of our second year involved learning the care of the medical and post-op surgical patient. Fourth floor of the hospital had a medical unit, plus pediatrics, fifth floor was medical, and sixth floor was surgical/orthopedic. The three floors were our clinical laboratory, where we did hands-on care.

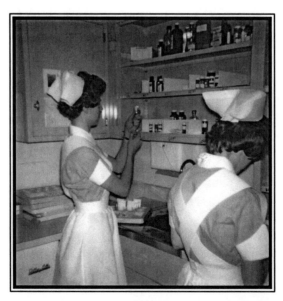

Vera Kemp, in the medication room, drawing up an injection.

On Tuesday, Wednesday, and Friday, we worked as students caring for assigned patients on the med/surg units. An instructor was always with us at these times. In the afternoons, we went to our med/surg class. Many times our lecturer was a physician.

Our instructors tried to find us patients that would coincide with what we were studying in our nursing classes. Sometimes that was possible, and other times it was not. It was very helpful to get our clinical assignments the day before in order to prepare for our patients and the disease processes that they had encountered. We did total nursing care for our assigned patients, including giving them a bath, medications, treatments, walking them, and keeping the bed and bedside in neat order. At first, we took care of one patient, and taking care of all these details seemed like a large job. I marveled at how the nurses on the floor could do all this, and more!

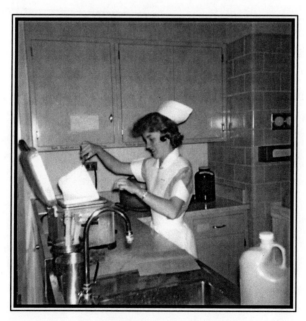

Jan Kmieciak working at the hot pack machine.

Half of the class had their surgery experience, while the other half was learning about medical patients. Then, we switched places.

We had gained a few tools to work with since that first awkward day when we were freshmen. Now we could put medical terminology to work, and at least we could figure out the body part that was affecting the patient. Having had the first surgery experience gave more experience tools to use, as well. And, we could draw from our nurse aide experience for some of the basic knowledge learned there.

In our med/surg classes, we studied the nursing care needed for various illnesses. Sometimes the instructor would begin with a review of the anatomy and physiology of the area involved in a particular disease. This was quite helpful, but when the doctors came to talk (bless them for doing so), many times they talked way over our heads. Once, I saw one of our nursing instructors roll her eyes when a physician was discussing the Kreb's cycle and how it affected a patient's recovery.

We'd come out of the classroom when class was over and say: "What was that all about?"

So, off to the dorm for a smoke or a coke and then hit the books. Our med/surg text was thick and devoid of pictures, so it was often hard to get into the process of reading. Somehow we came to understand what was required and we were able to pass any tests.

There was always so much to learn, and there never was quite enough time to thoroughly get into the material. Again, we went through every body system and learned not only the disease process, but the nursing care, medications to treat the disease, and patient prognosis.

Part of our instruction included pre- and post-op care. The pre-op checklist was strictly adhered to; not one part could be overlooked before sending a patient to surgery. Nail polish removed? Check! Patient voided? Check! ID band in place? Check! The operating room nurse came to the unit and reviewed the checklist prior to taking the patient to surgery. It had better be correct or surgery would be delayed. In surgery, things moved like a well-oiled clock.

Mrs. Terhaar was an instructor on sixth floor, the surgical unit. She was a tall, thin woman with very dark hair, and she rarely had a smile on her square-jawed face. She spoke in a twangy monotone voice that put me to sleep during her lectures. My notes from her lecture, many times, showed a squiggly line as I had nodded off.

During clinical, we never knew where Mrs. Terhaar might be lurking. One morning, behind drawn privacy curtains, I was doing a patient bed bath. I noticed large shoes under the curtain, and then I saw Mrs. Terhaar's peaked nursing cap towering above the curtain. I was startled for a moment when I saw her hand creep in between the two drawn curtains. I could hear no words uttered from her lips as she extended her finger into the basin bath water sitting on the bedside stand. Perhaps she thought I wouldn't see her. It turned out that this was her method to check the bath water temperature.

One day, Mrs. Terhaar became very exasperated with me during clinical. I don't remember why, but I do remember what she said: Miss Ukura, you cain't put a pillar in a pillarcase!
—Carolyn Ukura Kuechle

Post-op care was learned on the surgical unit with patients who had experienced many different types of surgeries. Each person was a unique individual with special needs, and for whom individualized care was given.

"Look at what the doctor did to me!" This was said by an anguished woman of about fifty, as soon as I stepped into her room. She was one of my first patients during my medical, post-surgical patient experience.

I approached the woman, who had had a colostomy performed the previous day. I uncovered her abdomen, while protecting her privacy, to look at the stoma (opening of the colon to the skin surface). There was a large ABD (gauze dressing) covering the surgical site and a plastic colostomy bag protruding underneath it. There was dark red drainage in the bag, and the dressing was dry. Her abdomen was enlarged, and I asked her about pain. She seemed to be more upset about the colostomy than in pain.

I felt very sorry for this patient, and I wondered how in the world I was ever going to take care of her. Then it dawned on me that we had learned about the concept of empathy. Many times, in our basic nursing classes, we had talked about empathy, a process of feeling with the patient rather than feeling for the patient. At first, I didn't quite understand how to do this, or why it was important. Now, all at once, I knew what they were talking about. I couldn't be of much help to this woman if all I did was to be sympathetic and sorry for her. My job was to help her regain her strength and to help her learn to care for herself.

I quickly checked the patient's vital signs, and then was off to find my instructor. She'd know what to do. Just as I was opening the door to leave, there was Mrs. Elvin! I was glad to see her (even though I felt she thought I'd never amount to much!). She came into the room, and we got the woman comfortable. Then Mrs. Elvin launched into great information for the patient about what to expect from her surgery. I was amazed, and wondered why I didn't know how to do what seemed to come so naturally to Mrs. Elvin. It was her voice of experience speaking to the patient, and I wondered if I'd ever be able to do what she had done. This was a great learning opportunity for me that I could put into my toolbox.

In our classroom work, we had learned that all patients needed to be prepared for the type of surgery they would be having, and they needed an understanding of what their post-op course would be like. It was stressed to us that the doctor would take care of explaining most of this to the patient. From what this patient had just said to me,

I wondered how much preparation she had been given. She would have many changes, from caring for the colostomy, to how she may feel about her body, to what clothing she could wear. I wasn't quite sure how to respond to what she was saying. I wanted her to learn to help herself, and I listened closely to what she was telling me. I tried to show her that I cared. I offered encouragement as we got her up in the chair for the first time after surgery, and as we took her for a short walk. I learned not to hurry her, but to offer reassurance that what she was about to do was possible.

Type 2 (adult onset) diabetes was an important but confusing disease process that we encountered in patients on the medical/surgical units. We learned about the many changes that could occur in the body as a result of having diabetes, especially untreated diabetes. At that time, there were very few oral drugs for treating diabetes. Therefore, insulin injection was more readily used for treatment. Urine glucose testing was the method used for diabetics to monitor their sugar levels. Signs and symptoms of low and high blood sugar and how to respond was critical. Then there was insulin. There were several different types of insulin available, and we had to learn the onset, peak, and duration of each type. Learning how to give the injection was another major learning opportunity. The importance of diet was a major situation in diabetes, as well. With all these many facets of diabetic care, it was easy to get them all mixed up, but with a test looming, we had better get this right!

Sometimes in our med/surg classes, Mrs. Elvin, who did the bulk of the lectures, had a strange way of expressing herself. She would say: "The patient might feel faint and have sweaty skin, and that type of a thing."

We always wondered what "and that type of a thing" really meant. As our classes progressed, she used this phrase over and over again, until we started keeping track of how many times she said it in one lecture. When we compared notes after class, no wonder we couldn't keep things straight!

While learning about the nursing care of the many patient illnesses, there were specific procedures taught and demonstrated. I'll never forget when Miss Haaland placed a naso-gastric tube through Mrs. Elvin's nose and threaded it through her esophagus into her stomach. Mrs. Elvin coughed, and her face turned red during this procedure! She was obviously quite distressed. How very dedicated a teacher she was to allow herself to be the patient in this demonstration for our benefit.

There were many principles learned that day. That this was an uncomfortable procedure for the patient being the main one. The importance of explaining the procedure before, and reassuring the patient during the procedure, were primary. Educating the patient regarding how this procedure could be very helpful in relieving abdominal distention in a variety of bowel conditions was also stressed. Some of us had the opportunity to perform this procedure during our nursing education. Others had to remember how it was done, read the printed hospital procedure, and gain assistance before doing this procedure when working as a registered nurse.

Occasionally, we had a movie during classroom time as another teaching method. It was quite a welcome change from the lecture format. During the ENT (ear, nose, and throat) unit, we saw a vivid and remarkable film. It showed the workings of the middle ear. The bones of the middle ear actually moved to the song "The Stars and Stripes Forever." It was quite fascinating to see the bones vibrating to the beat of that classic song!

A short class on diet therapy, taught by a dietician, was included during this semester. She stressed the importance of nutrition in a patient's treatment and recovery. We had certain tasks we had to accomplish during this learning experience. One of the tasks was to time how long it took for a patient's tray to get from the dietary kitchen to the patient's bedside. I had a problem with understanding the importance of that.

Maybe it was because I worked on 5B-medical, in the student work program, that I came to enjoy medical nursing. Many of the patients were chronically ill and older, and it seemed to me that this was a more relaxed kind of nursing. Not being very crisis oriented, or tech oriented, this fit me better. Our patients had all the usual afflictions of diabetes, heart, lung, kidneys, etc., but one lady stands out from the rest. She was an older lady, quite obese, and both of her legs were enormous, hard, and deformed. She had lymphedema, a blockage in the lymphatic system preventing lymph fluid from draining well, causing the swelling in her legs. But, hers was the worst kind; it was called elephantiasis. She had much difficulty walking, and she was mostly chair bound. What I remember about her was her smile and positive attitude, in spite of having such a large burden in life. Sometimes, it is the patient who is the greatest teacher.

—Carolyn Ukura Kuechle

This was a semester of wide experiences and learning that could be applied to every age of patient. In clinical, we gained confidence in assessing patients while applying book learning to the real situation.

In that era, nurses did not listen for bowel sounds, check for distention (palpate the abdomen), or do much patient education. Today's nurse does this and much, much more! Today's nurse must also have adeptness with technology and be able to advance as the changes in technology advance. And, with the many changes, she or he must also be a compassionate teacher. Today, nursing has branched out into many specialty areas, with most nurses working in specific areas of nursing.

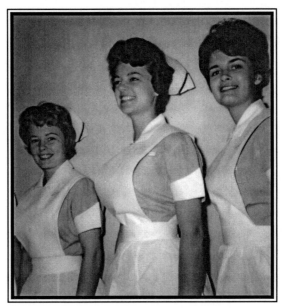

Black stripe on cap distinguishing senior status.
Sandra Morrow, Vicki Lymburner, and Barbara Carlson.

CHAPTER 17

Northwest to Alaska

By: Carolyn Ukura Kuechle

After a challenging nearly two years of H. Joan's very focused goal of trying to make proficient nurses and "ladies" out of us, Betty, ever on a quest, began to think of a new adventure, a freedom to be experience during the 1963 summer. Before long, she had enlisted her roommate, Vera, me, and after some hesitation, Karen, to join her. After the many rules and regulations encountered at the nursing school, we yearned to be in a less restrictive situation, at least for the summer. We were looking for a totally new experience, thinking how fun it would be to have the freedom to actually chew gum and sit with crossed legs. Proper behavior as advised in H. Joan's "make ladies out of them" class had us merely sit with ankles crossed, no gum chewing, and our hands folded in our lap. Of course, that was not the official title of the class, but it was her focus, nonetheless.

Betty began writing letters to hospitals in several states to inquire about possible summer employment. After receiving several letters of rejection, it wasn't looking very hopeful for our summer adventure. It seemed no one wanted us. And then, an exciting turn of events occurred! February 18, 1963, a letter from Sister Mary Clarita, the director of nursing service at Saint Ann's Hospital in Juneau, Alaska, arrived. In the letter she expressed that she not only wanted, but she seemed enthused, about us. She invited us to Juneau for the summer to work at their small community hospital. Sister Clarita included application blanks for employment.

This was exciting! Alaska, really! None of us had ever traveled much farther than across the Minnesota/Iowa or Minnesota/Wisconsin borders, except Betty, who was born in South Dakota. We knew nothing about Alaska, other than some of the typical stereotypes we had heard of beautiful scenery, gold prospecting, and grizzly bears. To work in Alaska was really above and beyond any imagining of where we could travel for the summer.

It took very little time to form an affirmative answer to Sister Clarita's invitation to work at Saint Ann's. We did the paperwork and sent it off to her. We were more than happy to accept the offer of summer employment, and we told her that we would travel as soon as the current school year was completed.

On February 27, 1963, an official employment acceptance letter arrived from the Sisters of Saint Ann. Included was information regarding the type of uniform we were expected to wear, hours of work, salary of $1.83 hourly, and housing information. A copy of the nurses' permanent rotating schedule spelled out exactly what our work schedule would be, and it was based on a seven-week rotation of day, evening, and night shifts. We would work seven shifts, and then have three days off. The bottom line of the nurses' permanent rotating schedule stated: "It is the fairest schedule ever known."

Though we had much to accomplish in the next three and a half months to complete the second year of our coursework, the excitement and planning for our Alaska summer adventure had begun! In discussions and research of how we would travel to Alaska, we settled on rail travel to Seattle and air to Juneau. We bought our train tickets and reserved our airline tickets.

Finally, at 11:00 a.m. the morning of June 13, 1963, we attended the last class of the second year of nursing school. We were free at last! In anticipation, Karen and I went grocery shopping to help fill our Styrofoam cooler for the train trip to Seattle. We paid for our plane tickets and did last minute things—we baked a chicken! And we packed.

Early on our departure date, June 14, 1963, Mrs. Vy Beard, Betty's mother, arrived at the dormitory to transport us to The Minneapolis Great Northern Railway Station. We took along one suitcase each, and an iced, packed Styrofoam cooler. After detailed planning for this adventure, and months of anticipation, the time to leave had finally arrived!

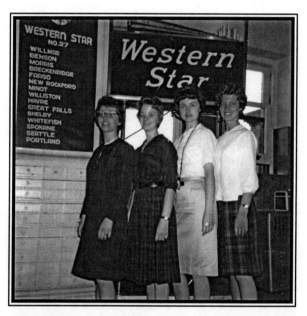

Beginning the journey: Karen Young, Carolyn Ukura, Betty Beard, and Vera Kemp.

At the railway station, we boarded a train called the Western Star. Although we were a bit nervous about heading out on our own that beautiful mid-June day, we climbed the steps into the train and never looked back. Before settling into our seats we, twice, made a grand tour of the train, including the Pullman section and the very plush lounge. We wouldn't be seeing the Pullman section again, as we had paid for a seat to sit in, and that was all. Nor would we be visiting the plush lounge. Our food supply for our journey west to Seattle, Washington, was stored in our coat pockets and the Styrofoam cooler.

After exploring the train, we settled into our seats, and soon the train pulled out of the railway station as Seattle beckoned us westward. We left the Twin Cities behind as we sped along the rails and watched the scenery out the large side windows. We traveled into western Minnesota, through North Dakota, and into eastern Montana, where fields of corn, wheat, flaxseed, barley, rye, and hay glistened in the sun and rippled from the wind as we moved along through the countryside. Farms and farm animals, then cattle ranches, sped on by.

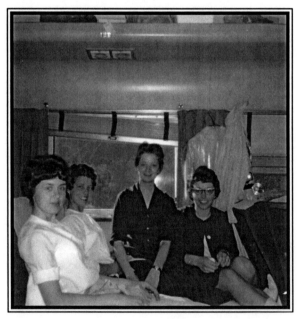

Sitting on the train: Betty Beard, Vera Kemp, Carolyn Ukura, and Karen Young.

The Western Star made many stops at the towns along the way. First it was Willmar, then on to Benson, Morris, and Breckenridge in Minnesota. In North Dakota, there were train stops at Fargo,

New Rockford, Minot, and Williston. We were allowed to get out of the train at various depot stops. Karen Young wrote, "At the depot stops, we got out of the train and walked around. We had about five minutes to buy ice cream."

Nightfall came. Besides ice cream, another expenditure was for a pillow. The cost was thirty-five cents per pillow, obtained from the porter. We slept on and off throughout the night, trying to get comfortable while sitting upright in our seats. Vera and Betty were seated directly behind Karen and myself.

As the train rumbled on into the early morning light, I waited with spirits soaring for the first glimpse of a mountain. We were traveling through Montana, heading to the towns of Havre, Great Falls, Shelby, and Whitefish, when I saw the foothills of the mountains in the distance!

As we got closer, the lofty ranges of the Rocky Mountains, with their high snowcapped peaks in irregular formations, stood with grandeur and majesty as the train came into Glacier National Park. The wide glaciers appeared to flow between some of the mountains tops while beautiful waterfalls cascaded down the mountainsides. Spruce and fir trees with their lush, green colors grew part way up the mountainsides. The wide and treacherous-looking Flathead River flowed alongside the railroad tracks. Having only seen the hills of Duluth, Minnesota, I was amazed to see the splendor and greatness of the Rockies out the train windows. I have never forgotten that moment.

After we left beautiful Glacier National Park behind, the train traveled into the town of Whitefish, Montana, a lovely place with mountains from every vista.

The train did not stop as we traveled through the shrub lands of the Columbia Plateau, which started with the small expanse of northern Idaho and into eastern Washington. My thought that Washington was lush and green was dispelled when I saw the brown, desert-like vegetation.

> After traveling for three days and two nights on the train, we arrived in Seattle at midnight. From the train depot, we took a taxi to the airport. I saw the Space Needle in the distance! We slept on couches in the airport. But, I didn't sleep. I watched the planes come and go, and the sun rise over Mount Rainier.
> —Karen Young Miller

At the airport, there were couches to rest on, and we slept a little. The couches were quite comfortable after sleeping upright in our train seats for two nights. We met eight University of Minnesota engineering students. They, too, were on summer adventures; three of the students were going to Juneau, Alaska. We visited with them as we waited for our 8:30 a.m. flight to Juneau.

None of the four of us had flown before, and it was with much excitement and apprehension that we boarded the Pan American World Airways airplane. We found our seats, settled in, and fastened our seat belts. After a short time, the door of the airplane was closed, and the plane began to taxi down the runway. It gained speed. It sped down the runway and lifted into the gray-colored sky!

Through torrents of rain, we descended into Ketchikan, Alaska. After a short time, we were back in the sky and on our way again. We experienced a bumpy ride to Juneau. As we flew, the rain fell hard against the airplane windowpanes. My stomach was in a knot as I caught glimpses through the fog and rain of looming mountains. I held my breath and closed my eyes as the plane circled. Would we ever be on the ground, or would we fly into a mountain? Finally, we began to descend through the rain and the fog. We had landed on the airport runway of the Juneau, Alaska, airport! We sighed a collective sigh of relief.

We had reached our long-awaited destination. With anticipation and enthusiasm undaunted, we gathered our belongings and exited the airplane. We hailed a taxi to take us the twelve miles into town. It was then that Vera realized she didn't have her return plane ticket. Back to the airplane she dashed, and very fortunately, underneath her seat she found her ticket!

Soon we had our first experience of Alaskan hospitality. Our female taxicab driver took us on a tour of the city, without extra fee, before we arrived at the Rochovich Apartment Building located on Basin Road. Sister Clarita had arranged for this to be our home for the summer. It was located one block up a steep hill from the hospital.

Lois Poole, our landlady, was not present to let us into our apartment upon our arrival. We soon met our neighbors, Saint Ann's nurses who lived in the apartment building. We left our belongings with them, and we excitedly made our first of many walks down the hill to Saint Ann's Hospital.

At the hospital, we found Sister Clarita, who very enthusiastically welcomed us to Saint Ann's! She wore the traditional habit of the sisters of Saint Ann, with only her sweet, angelic face showing from under her veil. She took us on a tour through the hospital while introducing us to the staff and patients. We sensed a relaxed, casual, and friendly atmosphere. Sister Clarita must have done some advanced cheerleading about our arrival, not just at the hospital, but about town, when people would say when we met them: "You must be the student nurses from Minnesota."

After our hospital visit, we walked back to the Rochovich Apartment Building. Our landlady had arrived, and she escorted us from the apartment building's front entrance to our small apartment located at the bottom of the long flight of stairs. The south wall of the building was on ground level, and there were two windows, one in the kitchen, and one in the living room/bedroom. Our three-room apartment was furnished. It was cozy, with a very tiny kitchen, one bedroom, and a small living room. The living room had a couch that became a bed, and it served as the second bedroom. Vera and Betty shared the bedroom, while Karen and I slept in the living room. We soon discovered that the bathroom shower had a drainage problem with usually about two inches of water standing in the bottom. The rent was $134 per month; utilities were extra.

Many of Saint Ann's nurses lived in the Rochovich Apartment Building. They were very friendly and helped us out when needed. They invited us to dinner, introduced us to their friends, and took us on outings. Some were Canadians, and a colloquialism they used to end a sentence was: "Aye?"

We unpacked, settled in, and wrote letters home that evening. After an exciting journey, and limited sleep of the past few days, we were off to sleep early on that June 16, 1963, night, in spite of the very long daylight hours.

At 7:45 a.m. the next day, we were up and dressed, and we had walked down the hill to Saint Ann's. We were ready and eager to learn about Saint Ann's, and to begin our hospital duties.

Saint Ann's Hospital was established in 1886 by three sisters: Sister Mary Zenon, Sister Mary Bon Secours, and Sister Mary Victor from Saint Ann's Convent in Victoria, British Columbia. The three sisters reached Juneau in the pouring rain on September 11, 1886. They walked down the plank from the ferry to be greeted by Father Althoff, the village priest. He led them up through the town by lantern light to the little frame house, which was to be the hospital. Two weeks later, they took in their first patient.

The sisters found a town, described by Senator Ernest Gruening as: "A struggling collection of cabins, of log and frame buildings, between which wound unpaved trails hardly recognizable as streets. It was a raw, rugged frontier."

Juneau, at that time, was a mining town, founded during the 1880 gold rush days. It was named after Joe Juneau, a prospector who had found gold in the area. Saint Ann's Hospital in 1963 was a combination of units constructed in 1913, 1917, 1933, and 1954. Sadly, in 1964, the sisters realized their building was inadequate as a hospital, and though they tried hard to obtain funding, Saint Ann's was scheduled to close as a hospital when a new hospital, built by the Greater

Juneau Borough, was to open in 1971. (And it did.) Subsequently, Saint Ann's became a nursing home.

The information in the preceding paragraphs are from *Southeast Alaska Empire*, dated Saturday, May 17, 1969.

Juneau is the capital city of the state of Alaska. It is inaccessible to the outside world except by airplane or boat, and it has one fifty-mile-long road. Surrounding the city on three sides are mountains and glaciers that tower above the city. It is a beautiful place with trees that grow tall and green, and waterfalls cascade down the mountainsides. Juneau is located on the Gastineau Channel, and Douglas Island is located directly across the channel. Secretary of State William H. Seward purchased Alaska in 1867 from Russia for $7,200,000. At the time, it was called Seward's Folly or Seward's Icebox. When the many natural resources of Alaska became known, Seward no longer was berated for his purchase. Alaska became the forty-ninth state in 1959.

The first people of the Juneau area were the "people of the tides," the Tlingit Indian tribes. For their sustenance, they had learned to rely on the ocean and the rivers for fish and seaweed and the land for hunting game and picking berries in the summer. They carved canoes out of cedar, set fish traps, and plucked fish out of the sea with spears and hooks. They were a sociable people and enjoyed a rich cultural life. They celebrated weddings, births, deaths, and other occasions with a potlatch that would go on for days. This was a festival celebrated with feast, music, dance, theater, and spiritual ceremonies. Everyone who attended was given a gift by the host family. The status of any given family is raised in Tlingit culture not by who has the most resources, but by who gives the most away.

A totem pole was usually part of the potlatch ceremony; its purpose was to commemorate people or special events. A totem pole is hand carved of wood in symbols of animals or spirits, and it has meaning that constitutes a story, legend, or myth.

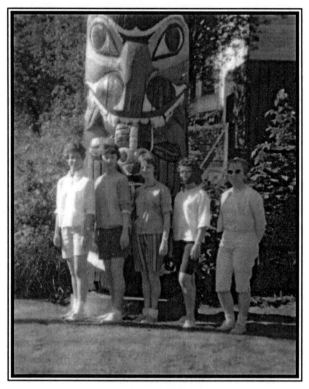

Standing by the totem pole in Downtown Juneau:
we four and our friend, Alice Green.

The Tlingit had lived in the Juneau area for many centuries, and they had never seen a white man until the mid-1700s when the Russians, and then the Spanish explorers, arrived. As with all the native cultures, their way of life drastically changed with the advent of the white man. In the nineteenth century, their cultural potlatch was outlawed by both the Canadian and United States governments.

Saint Ann's was a seventy-eight-bed hospital with twelve bassinets. The women and men were segregated by floor. Third floor was the woman's floor. It included the nursery, labor, and delivery rooms. Second floor was the men's floor. It also included pediatrics and the emergency room. Pharmacy, laboratory, x-ray, operating rooms, and administrative offices were located on the first floor. The lower floor consisted of the main kitchen, dining rooms, and laundry. Since we frequently ate meals at the hospital, we know the food served at Saint Ann's was home cooked and delicious!

After the first "get acquainted" day at Saint Ann's, we settled into our hospital routine. Betty was assigned to the women's floor and the nursery, while Vera and I worked the men's floor and pediatrics. Karen worked in all areas.

> I believe it was one of my first shifts in labor/delivery, and our patient was a Native American mother-to-be. I had no experience in obstetrics, and I hadn't ever seen the birth of a baby. It was with great sadness for the mom, and for all of us helping her, that the baby was delivered stillborn.
> —Karen Young Miller

We worked all shifts (days, evenings, and nights) and extra shifts when needed. If it was very busy or short staffed at the hospital, one of the four who was on duty ran up the hill to the apartment to get help! Since we had no telephone at the apartment, it wasn't a matter of ignoring a ringing telephone. No, you couldn't ignore that person who was calling your name and shaking you from your slumber. It was get up, speedily get ready for work, and be off down the hill to Saint Ann's.

> According to the Alaska natives, the summer of 1963 was sunnier and dryer than most Juneau summers, but we still experienced lots of rain. With our umbrellas up, we walked along in the rain, going up and down the hill to the hospital, singing the Johnnie Ray hit of the '50's, "Just Walkin' in the Rain."
> —Karen Young Miller

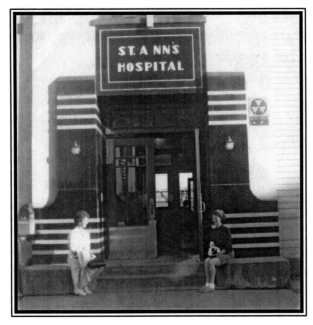

In front of Saint Ann's: Vera Kemp and Carolyn Ukura.

Betty was assigned the job of making the infant formula when she worked the night shift. This was quite an arduous task, and she went a half hour early on her own time to do it. There were several ingredients that had to be mixed together and put into sterile bottles for the infant feedings. She said: "I don't know how anyone can properly make the formula without extra time to do it!"

It wasn't very often that all four of us were home or off-duty together. Usually there was at least one of us at home sleeping, having worked the night shift or a double shift.

At Methodist we were used to everything being modern and at our fingertips. At Saint Ann's, we wheeled the oxygen tank and suction machine into the patient room. The hot pack machine was down the hall in a utility room. Medications were dispensed from a cupboard at the nurses' station; there was not a separate medication room. Even so, Saint Ann's offered us a very rich and diversified learning experience.

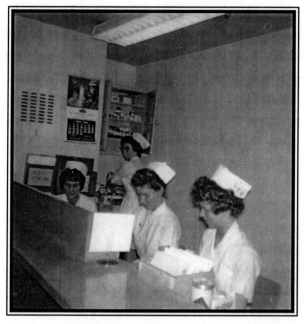

Second floor nurse's station.

Most Saint Ann's patients had the usual type of illness or injury that we had seen at Methodist Hospital in Saint Louis Park, Minnesota. What we hadn't seen at Methodist were injuries suffered by fishermen working the commercial fishing boats. Most of these injuries occurred when the fisherman got entangled in the boat's winch that was used to haul in the fishing nets from the sea. Many of these men had suffered multiple injuries and were in the hospital for several weeks. We learned to care for a person in traction with neck and back injuries, and how to work with a person who had casts on more than one extremity.

I had a young man who was my patient at the hospital. I remember walking into his room very cheerful-like and telling him I needed to set him up for traction because of his back problem. He said he didn't think he needed it. I said, "Oh yes, it's for you."

So, I applied the green, sticky, perforated strips to his legs as part of the traction procedure. After finding out I had put them on the wrong patient, I had to go back in his room to tell him. I then had to remove all those green, sticky, perforated strips off his hairy legs! Poor guy! The pain had to be unbearable. And, he was so kind to me about it all.

—Vera Kemp Germain

The pediatric unit contained about six beds and several cribs at the end of a wing on second floor. We cared for many babies under one year old. We were asked, if the patient count was low, and we weren't that busy, to go to the peds unit and just "Hold the babies." This was something we didn't mind doing at all.

A procedure that I had not seen previously involved giving subcutaneous fluid to a child for rehydration. This was done with very large needles that were injected into a three-year-old girl's thighs. This method seemed to work, but I did not see such a procedure after that.

A long remembered, and very special, patient whom we cared for on second floor was Roy Noland. He had been a sourdough at the turn of the century, and he had come to Alaska to pan for gold during the days of the gold rush. He was in his eighties in 1963, and he told stories from those days. He said he had never really struck it rich, but he had successfully panned gold. He never married and had no children. He'd had his leg amputated due to diabetes, and his stump site was not healing well. There was time to visit during his dressing changes. His favorite term for us was "cheechako." This was a term from the gold rush days meaning tenderfoot, greenhorn, or newcomer.

Roy and I corresponded after I left Juneau, and then I didn't hear from him any longer. I found out that he had died. I cherish a beautiful, hand-painted dish with a winter scene of an Alaskan food cache that he sent for a wedding present.

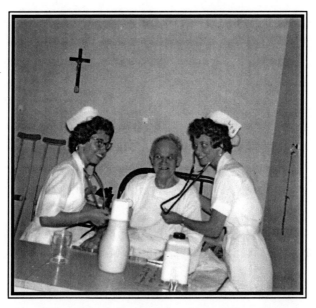

Ray Noland with Karen Young and Vera Kemp.

Another man in his fifties had recently had a heart attack, and he talked constantly. The treatment back then was that the cardiac patient had to stay in bed at all times with very restricted activity. The inactivity was causing him anxiety, and it was making him very fearful. He required a lot of reassurance. One day he said: "I'm afraid if I stop talking, I will die!"

This man did well, despite the treatment and inactivity.

Many of the patients at Saint Ann's were flown in from the surrounding geographic area. Saint Ann's took care of all possible medical problems, including alcohol-related situations.

One day I was caring for a patient with delirium tremors. The man was lying on his bed talking incoherently and picking things out of the air. This was a corner room, and it had a beautiful view of the Gastineau Channel with the mountains and glaciers beyond the channel. I turned away from the patient and stood before the unscreened, partially open window, and looked at the view. Suddenly, I sensed that he was right behind me. I turned around as he was putting his hands on my waist. He was very confused, and I was very startled! I took his hand in mine and talked to him as I led him away from the window. Fortunately, he calmly followed and went back to his bed without incident.

An eye-opener for me was working with an alcoholic with delirium tremors (DTs) who had become very confused and belligerent. I had never worked with anyone at Methodist in this kind of situation. We restrained him in his bed to keep him from hurting himself, or another person. Having to use a restraint on a patient was difficult for me.
—Karen Young Miller

One night Vera finished second shift, and she walked up the hill to our apartment building. She walked down the flight of stairs to our apartment, unlocked the door, and entered. In the window that was directly across from the door stood a man looking in the window! Upon seeing her, he quickly left. I had worked the day shift, and I was sleeping in my bed that was less than two feet away from the window.

Vera woke me from a very deep sleep to tell me about the man she had just seen looking in the window. Bolted awake, I jumped out of bed! Looking for a weapon, I grabbed the umbrella that was standing in the corner and headed for the door that led up the stairs and out of the apartment. With knees shaking and teeth rattling, I opened the door, and said: "I'm getting out of here."

Of course, Vera, in spite of the situation, thought it was quite comical to see me grab the umbrella and head for the door clad only in my white baby doll pajamas. She exclaimed: "No, no. Stay here. Don't go out there!"

By this time, I was awake and had an awareness of what I was doing. I turned around, came back into the apartment, and placed the umbrella back into the corner.

We stood by the window looking out, but we did not see the man. Another residential building was about fifteen feet from our building. Though it was dark outside, we could look into the uncovered window of an apartment in that building. The lights were on, and lying on the table by the window was a handgun, which only added to our fear.

After all that, it took awhile to get to sleep that night. Did that man know I was asleep on the bed just a few feet away from the window? And, fifty years later, I'm not certain if that window was closed or partially open. Did Vera's returning home at that time save me from an uncertain disaster? I can only say that it gave me the "shudders" when I thought of it. We never knew who the man looking in the window might have been, or who the people were who owned the gun that was left lying on the table.

The friendliness and hospitality of the Alaskans was very impressive! Their way of life was casual, relaxed, and oriented toward the outdoors.

> What I remember and liked about Alaska, and its people—there weren't the social classes like at home. The rich, middle, and poorer people were all together. Lawyers, doctors, workers, fishermen—they didn't have the elite club only. All people were one.
> —Karen Young Miller

Fishing was a frequent activity by the people of Juneau, and they shared their bounty. Fresh delicious salmon was a delicacy at our small table in the Rochovich apartment. Hunting was another outdoor activity enjoyed by many people, mainly men, living in Juneau. We were invited to dinners of moose meat and mountain goat, a new food experience, and always tasty.

Speaking of men, there were lots and lots of men in Juneau. We received invitations to go boating, fishing, hiking, dancing to

Dreamland, the Baranoff Bubble Room in the Baranoff Hotel, Mike's Place in Douglas, Occidental Bar, or to their homes for dinner, with some of the Saint Ann's nurses. Juneau offered many opportunities for social life and activity!

One night a fellow, who was interested in Vera, came by. I was the only one still dressed; the other three were already in their pajamas. They had rushed into the bedroom when they heard the knock on the door, and they stayed giggling in the bedroom while I ended up visiting with him for an hour before he finally gave up and left. Obviously, athletic Vera, with her infectious smile, pretty blue eyes, and curly hair, was not interested in seeing this fellow.

Karen and Betty went on a mountain climbing excursion with U of M engineers, Jim and Dave, whom we had first met at the Seattle airport. They carried a knapsack with their lunch in it and a large blade to ward off bears! After hiking many miles on the Mendenhall trail through mud and falling rocks, they reached the top of Mendenhall Glacier. It was quite windy and cold, with the wind blowing off the glacier, but the view was spectacular! My borrowed camera from my cousin Dick Ukura, that Karen carried, somehow fell into a glacial crevice as they walked on the glacier. Fortunately, they were able to retrieve it, but the camera was never quite the same, even after repair. After eating lunch, they started back down the trail. Returning to the end of the trail, they found they had no ride home! None of us seems to remember how they arrived at Mendenhall Glacier, but they hitchhiked the seventeen miles back to Juneau. Hitchhiking was common at that time, and it turned out to be part of our Juneau adventure.

The only one of us who experienced a fishing excursion was Karen, when she went out in Herb Olander's boat, the Sea Rake, with Herb, Don Stitchler, and Bev Connolly. It happened one gorgeous July day on beautiful Auke Lake. They fished for nine hours and Karen brought fish home. She had caught four salmon: two silvers, a king, and a chum weighing nine to eleven pounds each!

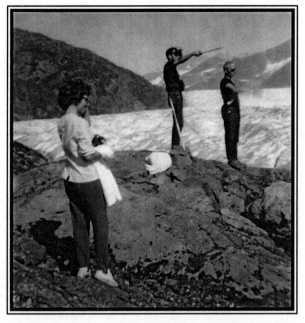

Mendenhall Glacier: Karen Young with Dave and Jim,
U of M engineering students.

The king fought for fifteen minutes. I got tired
and silly, and my belly was sore from the rod poking
it. My arm was ready to fall off from continually reel-
ing, causing me quite an ordeal. Got it, though!
—Karen Young Miller

The Perseverance Trail entrance to Mount Roberts was across
the street (Basin Road) and a few steps up from the Rochovich Apart-
ments. We took advantage of our quick "get away to the trail" where
we enjoyed many hikes. It was a three-mile hike to the old Perseverance Mine, where gold had been mined until 1944.

The trail was wide and easy to walk. There was lots of vegetation that included wildflowers, bushes with berries, and devil's club, a
rather nasty, tall, large-leafed plant growing along the trail sides. The
views were spectacular! Beautiful waterfalls cascaded down the sides

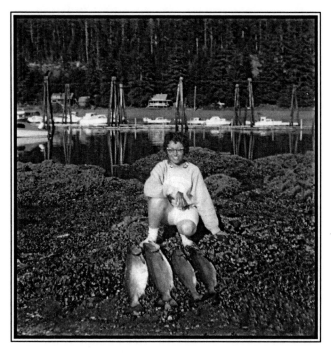

Karen Young and the four salmon that she caught!

of the mountains, Gold Creek ran fast, and there were other mountain streams that tumbled down the mountainsides. Looking upward,
we saw the beautiful white-blue of the glaciers and the white snow on
the mountaintops. The snow was melting from the warmth of the sun,
creating the rushing waterfalls and creeks. Sometimes, we just stood
there to survey, and take in, all the natural beauty that surrounded us
on Perseverance Trail.

In the beginning, Perseverance Trail had been used by the native peoples for mountain goat hunting, fishing, and berry picking. In
the 1880s, it became the first road in Alaska after gold was found in
the Silver Bow Basin by Joe Juneau and Richard Harris.

Since we were a group of "cheechakos," the Alaskans felt we
needed some guidance in living our lives in Juneau. They advised us
to make lots of noise to scare any bears nearby when hiking. They
told of a man in the previous summer, who had been attacked by a

grizzly. His skull was torn, and he was blinded. Also, there was a teenager whom we often saw downtown with a scarred face. He had been mauled by a bear.

We took the Alaskans' guidance very seriously. Whenever we hiked Perseverance Trail, we sang and shook cans with rocks in them. One of our favorite songs was "The Happy Wanderer." We never directly encountered a bear, but one day in the distance, we saw two grizzlies. They were on a mountain meadow above the path where we were walking.

Zach Gordon, a very kindly, older gentleman, had formed a teenage club in an old converted school in downtown Juneau. Probably through Sister Clarita, we were introduced to him, and he invited and encouraged us to attend the teenage club. Zach had a Ping-Pong table and a juke box that he provided quarters for us to play its records. Many of the kids who came to the club were male, and much younger than we. We played Ping-Pong with them and danced to the music of the jukebox. On our first visit, a fellow asked Betty to dance, and probably due to a shortage of females, we all danced a rather strange circle dance where we jumped up and down! Zach was always happy when any of us showed up at the teenage club.

Another activity that Zach involved us in was his Monday night discussion groups. They were held at various locations. Many times, they were held twelve miles from Juneau at Mendenhall Glacier Observatory, a lovely spot with large windows to look out at beautiful Mendenhall Glacier. This was a forum for the local young people, as well as for the many summer visitors, to meet and form friendships. Zach kept track of where the visitors were from, and he said as many as seventy-five different colleges, universities, and schools had been represented during that summer's discussion groups.

I usually felt the discussions were way above my head. The first discussion topic I attended was, "Are We Spoiling Our American Women?" Now, this was an interesting discussion from a mainly male point of view. It was mostly males who attended, and the discussions tended to be quite intellectual. I doubt in today's world, in most circles, that topic would even be an agenda item.

Other discussion topics were conformity, my own personal God, overpopulation, and segregation. Ever trying to keep us involved and coming to the discussion groups, Zach nominated us as discussion leaders. Vera and I led the discussion on overpopulation, where I said I wanted to have six kids. Although always kind, the other participants must have gotten a good chuckle over that one.

Zach tried very hard to make our Juneau summer interesting. He told us he would like to interview us to be on the local radio station. Zach did a radio show to promote his teenage club, Monday night discussion groups, people of Juneau, the many summer visitors, and local areas of interest. On the appointed day and time, he came to Saint Ann's, where he interviewed and taped us, along with Sister Mary Clarita. We talked about our school of nursing, how we came to work at Saint Ann's, our thoughts on the discussion groups, and our Juneau experience. He gave us a copy of the tape to take home. In listening to the tape many years later, I thought we sounded quite stiff and formal.

Then, Zach had us meet the sailors, but not all 1,500 of them at one time. The USS Bennington, an aircraft carrier, was docked at Auke Bay. Juneau was swarming with sailors, and I don't think they let all of them off the ship at the same time. Zach invited us to come to the teenage club where we met many, many sailors. Our friend, Alice Green from Eugene, Oregon, who went on many adventures with us, came along.

We four, Alice, and six sailors went on a hike up Perseverance Trail and to the mine. The sailors were funny and enjoyable. However, unbeknownst to us, one of the sailors had brought along a bottle of liquor that he was sipping. He became troublesome for the other five sailors who were with us. With that turn of events, we decided to hike back down the mountain. By this time, the trail and the mountain were swarming with sailors. We met many along the way. A whole mountainside of sailors became rather intimidating, and we were quite happy when we got back in our apartment.

Our last Zach-inspired adventure was on August 21, 1963, when he had us meet William A. Egan, the state of Alaska's first and then current governor, at the governor's mansion. The governor did not seem particularly enthused or talkative, and Zach did most of the talking. We were quite embarrassed when none of us knew who was Minnesota's governor! Due to a very close race, there had been a Minnesota vote recount that had lasted 139 days. In March 1963, it was known that Karl Rolvaag had beaten Governor L. Anderson by only ninety-one votes in this extremely close election. We obviously hadn't been paying attention to the local news of the day in 1963. We had our photo taken with Zach and Governor Egan, but we never saw it.

Zach Gordon was a lawyer from Pennsylvania who had come to Juneau during WWII to direct the USO Club. He hosted hundreds of servicemen stationed in Juneau, as well as those en route to different war zones. After the war, he remained in Juneau and convinced the community to convert the USO facilities into a teenage club. He lived simply, and was a tireless worker for the teenage club. Though he died in 1977, the teenage club, now known as the Zach Gordon Youth Center, carries on in Juneau.

The local pub and landmark, The Red Dog Saloon, was located downtown. It held quite a fascination with us for its unusual and unique decor. There were many Alaskan artifacts, including muskets, a bearskin rug, snowshoes, moose antlers, animal heads, traps, a totem pole, and other memorabilia hanging on the walls. We made several trips downtown to "check it out." By that I mean we would stand inside the swinging doors and observe the happenings. Though Vera and Betty had turned twenty-one, neither Karen nor I were of age to be in the bar. The Red Dog Saloon was reminiscent of the gold rush days of 1898. We entered through swinging doors, and there was sawdust spread over the floor. The bartenders wore red and white striped vests, while pouring drinks with both hands. It had an upright piano standing in the corner, and seventy-three-year-old "Ragtime Hattie" was the piano pounder! Above the piano was a large sign that read: Red Dog Saloon, Hattie, Queen of

Ragtime, Juneau, Alaska. In addition to spirits consumed, there was lots of spirited dancing and singing that occurred at the Red Dog Saloon!

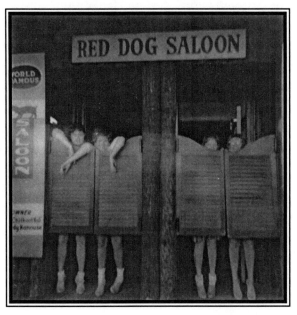

Standing inside the swinging doors of the Red Dog Saloon.
(L) to (R): Betty Beard, Vera Kemp,
Carolyn Ukura, and Karen Young.

July 4, 1963, turned out to be a lovely, sunny, summer day in Juneau. Karen and I had worked the day shift, and after work, she and I and Bev Connolly, a nurse from Saint Ann's, walked downtown. There was a navy destroyer docked in the harbor downtown, and once again, there were many sailors around town. Civilians were being allowed to visit the ship, so we climbed up and onto the deck of the destroyer. Standing on the deck of that vessel, we got a feel for how it might be to travel the ocean blue on a calm sea, as well to imagine "rocking and rolling" when the weather had turned stormy and the sea tumultuous.

At the time, I didn't think of how these contrasts compare to life itself. All is very calm, and in a moment's time, our lives can become unpredictable and stormy.

Bev took us out to eat at Percy's and we went
to the movie *Ice Palace*. After that, we went to see the
Fourth of July fireworks at a small boat harbor with
Herb and Brida. The fireworks were very pretty with
the full moon showing behind the mountain.
—Karen Young Miller

One morning, Betty and I were home when there was a
knock on the door. We opened the door, and who should be standing
there, but Vy and Bob Beard, Betty's parents. They had come all the
way from Princeton, Minnesota! They were not known to do much
traveling, and Betty was totally shocked to see them standing there.
Mr. Beard, with his dry sense of humor, entertained us, but unfortunately, he developed a respiratory infection and was ill for most of the
time they were with us. They stocked our refrigerator, and Mrs. Beard
cooked for us. We were able to take them to Mendenhall Glacier and
the Shrine of Saint Therese with Alice Green and her friend, Royal.
We enjoyed their five-day visit.

Alas, all comes to an end. On August 27, 1963, we were
packed and waiting in our apartment for our friend, Herb Olander,
to take us to Auke Bay. Many Alaskan friends had advised us to turn
in our return airline tickets and instead to travel via ferry down the
Inside Passage of southeast Alaska to Prince Rupert, Canada, and
ride the remaining distance via rail. And actually, we hadn't needed
to think about this suggestion for very long after remembering the
bumpy plane ride we had experienced when flying into Juneau. This
turned out to be very good advice, as we enjoyed a scenic ferry ride of
southeast Alaska and a train ride through beautiful British Columbia!

Herb hadn't arrived, and we felt we couldn't wait any longer to
arrive in Auke Bay to board the 3:00 a.m. Alaska state ferry, the Taku.
So, we had called a taxi. We closed the door to our apartment for the
last time, and we were loading our belongings into the taxi when Herb
arrived. He had gotten involved with his fish-smoking project, and he

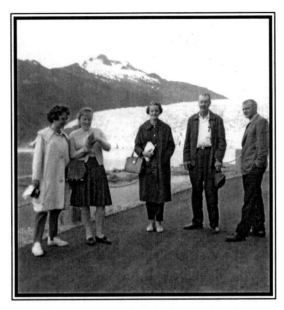

Karen Young, Alice Green, Vy and Bob Beard,
and Royal, Alice's friend, as they stood on the walkway
to the Menenhall Glacier Visitor Center.
Mendenhall Glacier is in the background.

had lost track of time. We said our goodbyes to Herb and had our last ride down Basin Road. It had been a great experience, and we were sad to leave, but we left with wonderful memories of Juneau, Alaska.

At Auke Bay, we boarded the Taku. We were on the observation deck of the ferry, where there were comfortable couches to sit or lie down, and we slept until 9:00 a.m. We awoke to a heavy fog. It soon lifted, showing beautiful scenery, with mountains on both sides of the wide channel. The Taku made several stops on its way down the Inside Passage. We slept overnight on the ferry and arrived in Prince Rupert, Canada, at 6:00 a.m., August 28th. It was foggy as we departed the Taku. We could see very little as we rode in a taxi to the Canadian National Railways train depot.

At the depot, we embarked a four-car train that traveled through beautiful British Columbia to Prince George, Canada. We had a layover of four hours in Prince George. We somehow found a hotel where we could take a tub bath! After eating in a cafe, we boarded the train and continued our journey. We arrived in Jasper, Canada, at 7:00 a.m., August 29th.

After riding the train all day, at 9:00 p.m., we stopped in Saskatoon, Canada, long enough so we could go for a walk. We were in Winnipeg at 8:30 a.m., and we transferred into a one-car train. On we went through the open farmlands along the United States/Canada border. It was quite a contrast to all the mountains we had seen in the west. We transferred trains again at Manitoba Junction in North Dakota. Soon, we were back in Minnesota. Betty got off the train in Saint Cloud, while Vera, Karen, and I traveled on to Minneapolis. Thus ended our wonderful, Alaskan summer adventure!

On the fourteenth of June in '63
    we four went on liberty.
By train we saw plains, mountains, and cattle
    as we crossed the country to Seattle.

Minnesota, our homeland, was loved dearly,
    but young hearts are adventurous early.
"To Alaska!" This exciting dream was coming true
    to the last frontier and beginning of new.

From Seattle to Juneau the jet went roaring
    the weather was turbulent, the clouds were pouring.
We caught glimpses of mountains, glaciers, and such.
    A "bumpy" ride, it was all too much!

Finally we landed. Oh, to be on ground!
    It was raining and cloudy, difficult to see around.
From the airport it was twelve miles to go
    and we were in the capital, Juneau.

We settled into a cozy, little home
      in the basement and without a phone.
The three little rooms were a humble domain
      the Rochovich apartment was its name.

The people were genuine, kind, and warm.
      We soon found they could be counted on.
The days were long, 12 midnight still light,
      the atmosphere quaint, very much a delight!

No matter what time of night or day
      you would find, at least, one earning her pay.
Saint Ann's was our place of employment
      many hours were spent there in work and enjoyment.

On a beautiful day with the sun brightly shining
      exploring where gold once had been in mining.
Ah, but look over yonder, a falls to behold.
      This even beats panning for gold!

Perseverance Trail worthy of its name
      brown bear and mountain goat are not tame.
"Let's make noise so they'll know we are here."
      Who wants to tangle with a grizzly bear?

There were mountains surrounding three sides of the town
      Vera and Karen climbed without a frown.
Oh, but look on the next top over there
      not even those two would chance a grizzly bear!

Betty and Carolyn, they didn't mind
        looked longingly at the sights from behind.
They sat on a tree stump here and there a while
        it seemed they had climbed many a mile.

The time passed on—
        soon summer was gone.
From that quaint town
        with mountains all aroun'.

We packed up and left
        but, we never would forget,
Saint Ann's, Sister Clarita, Zach Gordon, and all.
        We had to return to finish our call.

We were so young,
        hadn't experienced life's run.
So much, so sure, we thought we knew.
        Years passed by, we hadn't had a clue!

For life leaves no soul,
        without experience to know.
Take the bad with the good,
        with purpose and joy understood.

Fifty years later, and
        the impact still greater.
For that was a summer, a fantastic summer,
        that Alaskan summer of '63!

                —Carolyn Ukura Kuechle
                (mostly written in 1963)

PART THREE

THE THIRD YEAR,
SEPTEMBER 1963

CHAPTER 18

Psychiatric Nursing at Hastings State Hospital

Life winds as a road, each step is a day;
Spirit a lamp that illuminates the way.

The road grows familiar, our steps become sure;
Landmarks of learning leave minds more mature.

—Author Unknown

It was the fall of 1963. We were seniors beginning our last year of nursing school. Psychiatric nursing, pediatrics, obstetrics, and newborns were the specialty areas that we were to experience in that year. It felt great to be in our last year—soon we'd be on our way in our chosen career! (For some of us, it just didn't seem like it was soon enough!) Half of us began the year with a three-month psychiatric rotation at Hastings State Hospital in Hastings, Minnesota, while the other half remained at Methodist Hospital.

Located at the juncture of the Mississippi and Saint Croix rivers, Hastings, Minnesota, is a scenic river town that formed in the 1850s. It has a rich, progressive history in taking advantage of its many resources to provide water power, shipping and milling, farming, as well as the arts. It is located about thirty-five miles from Methodist Hospital. We were on our own in finding transportation to and from Hastings.

We traveled into the town of Hastings via Highway 61 and made a left turn past a lovely old mansion. Crossing a suspension bridge, we drove up a hill to get into the Hastings State Hospital campus. We were told that a young female patient on suicide watch had recently ended her life by jumping from the suspension bridge. This was an introduction into the reality of psychiatric nursing.

Many beautiful hardwood trees grew throughout the campus. The hospital was comprised of Tudor Revival Architecture buildings that housed the patients, male and female, separately. Each building had three floors called "wards." Larger buildings included the education and administration buildings, and some were connected by underground tunnel. We observed the patients walking freely about the campus on the many concrete walkways.

Hastings State Hospital opened in 1900 as the Hastings Asylum for the Insane. It was built as a solution of what to do with people who were seen as defective or insane. This included people with mental illness, physical and mental disabilities, dementia, chemical dependency—all those categories of people not considered to be "normal." The intent was to isolate and protect society from them. The state hospital became a place for the admitted person to be taken care of and to live out their life. (Nick Ferraro, "History Project Tells Stories of Life at the Old Hastings State Hospital," *Pioneer Press*, January 31, 2012, http://www.twincities.com/ci_19864395.)

In 1963, and before we arrived for our three-month tenure at Hastings State Hospital, the 460-acre dairy farm had closed. Previous to its closing, the patients had produced garden and dairy products for the hospital.

Many of the patients whom we saw walking about the campus had been institutionalized for many years. They had acquired an "institutional look," perhaps due to not having the influence or stimulus of living with their families or of being out in the world. Except for the staff, most did not have visitors. Many had been put into the hospital and forgotten. At that time, there were no available resources for families in caring for their afflicted family members.

Through the years, many of the patients had been buried in the Hastings State Hospital/Asylum Cemetery located on state-owned land near the hospital. Only a number, but no name, marked their burial spot. Recent efforts have been made to identify and provide a granite marker for all these many people.

During the sixties, mentally ill people were usually treated at regional state hospitals, since there were very few psychiatric units in hospitals. Only mild cases of mental illness were treated in a clinic setting. The long-term institutionalized and the shorter-term (six months or so) were all treated in this setting. Mental illness had been, and still is, somewhat of a mystery to diagnose and treat. Medication for the treatment of mental illness became available in the mid-fifties with the drug Thorazine. Thorazine, Stelazine, and Compazine, major tranquilizers and antipsychotics, were drugs that were given patients on a regular schedule during our tenure at Hastings State Hospital.

So, this was the world we entered when we reported directly to the dormitory building at Hastings State Hospital on September 8, 1963. We were given a Spartan, private room containing a single bed, closet, desk, and chair. Each of us was given a set of keys, and the door to our room was to be kept locked. This, in itself, seemed rather "eerie." Like the dorm at Methodist, there was a community bathroom and shower. Once again, we unpacked our belongings and prepared for what lay ahead.

Mrs. Stewart, our housemother, looked over us. She seemed to be more fun and livelier than those at Methodist. Maybe it was because she didn't have Miss Barber lording over and putting the fear of God in her.

Our instructions were to report Monday, September 9th, to the education building. We donned our student nurse uniforms and had breakfast in the employee café, where we were served by hospital patients learning job skills. Here the meals were free. They weren't the finest, but they were free!

> The education building was locked when we arrived, so we lined up outside it. I stood there talking to one of my classmates when I suddenly felt this strange feeling in my hair, and I realized there was someone very near me. I turned to see a small man, who we later found out to be 'Walter.' He had been trying to stroke my hair. I was scared out of my liver! I'd never been approached in such a way. Walter stood there with his head down. He wore an ill-fitting, stained jacket, and he continually moved his thumbs across the palms of his hands. He looked very sad.
>
> Just then, the door opened to the ed. building. We were saved! Hurriedly, we walked up the steps into the classroom where our instructors, Miss Powers and Mrs. Olson, waited for us.
>
> After telling the instructors about the just-experienced hair touching, the socially acceptable shaking of hands was explained as the approach to use with Walter. It turned out that Walter had pulled this stunt with many of the new students who came to the hospital. And, there had been many before us.
> —Jan Kmieciak Stenson

We were given orientation and taken on a tour. They informed us that we could wear just our dress uniform, no white apron over it. That was great! We wore our caps, and the smokers could smoke with the patients on the unit. We all were given small boxes of wooden matches to light patient cigarettes, since no patient was allowed to carry matches. Our key ring included a key to the locked intensive care unit that was located in the administration building. The men's ward is where we would learn about long-term care in the psych setting. We would mainly work and experience the men's ward, as well as the locked intensive care unit, during our stint at Hastings.

Half of us went to the locked intensive care unit, and the rest went to the men's ward for clinical. After six weeks, we switched. We were given a male case study assignment while in the men's ward. First, we delved into the patient history and disease process. After meeting our patient, and spending one-to-one time trying to develop trust, we hoped to develop a relationship. This wasn't easy, as most of the patients did not want, or seemed unable, to verbally communicate. After all the information gathering, we wrote a report.

> I remember my case study (I think it was a six-week study). My patient's name was Carl, and he had severe schizophrenia. Carl had not uttered a word for years, and he spent most of his days pacing back and forth. My assignment was to try to develop some type of relationship/trust with Carl. So every day, all I did was walk alongside him, back and forth, back and forth. I was there for him, day in and day out—not chattering, but only listening and observing. As the days and weeks went by, I could tell by his eyes that he was waiting for me to come to walk with him.
>
> The greatest reward was when he gave me a very small smile, and he spoke a word or two. . . . I guess it was mission accomplished. He taught me about persistence, being quiet and listening, and just being there for someone.
> —Karen Young Miller

The next day we were on the wards. The intensive care ward being a locked unit presented the first opportunity to use the key in opening the heavy metal door to enter within. Walking into the space, it looked quite dreary, and rather untidy. The walls were plain and grayed. There was a small nursing station with charts, a medication room, and a few desks and chairs. The unit housed about twenty patients. There were two treatment rooms and a few offices where doctors could privately talk to their patients, review their charts, and write orders. There was a room called the "quiet room," and it was used for seclusion when a patient "acted out." This meant the patient had lost behavioral control and could be a danger to himself/herself or others.

At the end of the hallway was a dayroom filled with leather covered and chrome chairs in various sizes. None of the "décor" was pleasing, and it looked like a mismatched rummage sale had taken place. The windows surrounding the room had metal grates over them for protection from being broken, so there could be no glass shards to use to self-harm or to harm others. Nor could a broken window allow an escape route. A few patients, dressed in street clothes, sat in the chairs. Some seemed to be vacantly staring off into space. Others paced the floor.

Our first assignment was to try to talk with some of the patients. It was difficult getting a person to talk since we were using closed-ended questions that could be answered with a yes or no. And the conversation went nowhere. This wasn't going to be easy, and the environment felt awkward and uncertain, which didn't help at all.

We spent our mornings in clinical on the wards. We addressed our patients by their first names, something we didn't do at Methodist. The patients were to refer to us as "Miss." The afternoons were spent in classroom learning, and being tested, of course. In the evenings we studied. A major focus was learning therapeutic communication. This involved observing and listening to the patient, learning their interests, and trying to engage her/him. We kept the focus on the patient and did not divulge any personal information. Nor were

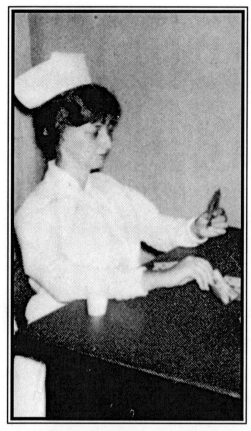

Mary Peterson playing therapeutic gin rummy on the ward.

we to get into any discussions of religion, politics, or sex. Freud's theories were the cornerstone for most psychiatric treatment back then, and the emphasis was on his theories and treatment.

Some preconceived ideas about a psychiatric hospital had been that we would see manic people literally swinging from the rafters and people in white coats putting straight jackets on them! This was not to be the case. Instead, we found the atmosphere to be rather quiet with people here and there; some of them were unkempt, many never made eye contact, and some had strange habits like moving their hands together in an odd fashion. We were to work in student pairs if we took our patients for walks outdoors, as a safety requirement.

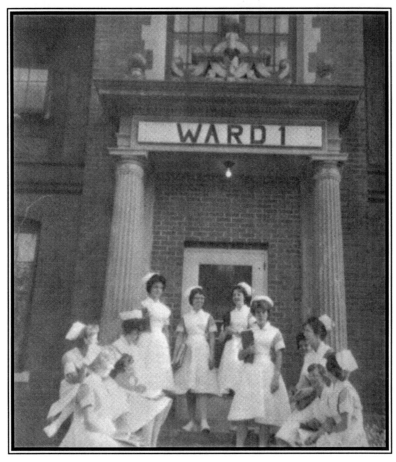

Standing outside Ward 1, September 1963.

We came to have some understanding of all the major mental illnesses, from anxiety to schizophrenia. There was not much discussion about drug therapy, since there were few drugs available for management of symptoms. Thorazine, Stelazine, and Compazine were used, though they tended to have lots of side effects. Electroconvulsive (ECT) therapy was used extensively, and we all saw patients having this therapy. (It was not a pretty sight.)

Electroconvulsive therapy looked dangerous and seemed almost like a Frankenstein movie, to think that passing electricity through a person's brain could be helpful. We were there to find out about these things, and once again we saw what we had barely heard of! When a patient was to have electroconvulsive therapy, it was performed in the intensive care unit. The patient was up and about and had to be nothing per oral (NPO) since midnight. The patients waiting to have ECT were usually anxious, and some of them paced the floors while waiting their turn.

The patient was brought into the treatment room where she/he climbed onto the exam table. A soft rubber device was inserted into the patient's mouth, and instructions were given to bite down on it. This was a type of mouth guard and airway. Electrodes were applied to the patient's temples by the psychiatrist. A staff nurse was instructed to push the current button when told to do so by the psychiatrist.

After receiving the electrical current through the electrode, the patient went into a grand mal seizure. This resulted in loss of consciousness, arching of the back, and body convulsing tightly for several seconds. He/she was held down by students, doctor, and other nurses for protection from injury or falling off the table. After a few minutes, the seizure ended. The patient relaxed and breathed deeply, sometimes with the aid of a mask and bag over his or her nose and mouth to deliver oxygen.

The patient was taken to a recovery room and observed closely for a half hour or so. Upon awakening, the person was very disoriented and couldn't remember time or place or what had occurred. Staying with the patient, we offered reassurance that he/she was all right and needed to rest for a while. After some of the immediate effects wore off, the person was ready to get up, but was closely observed for falling. Within a few hours, orientation had returned, along with the ability to resume prior activities.

The electroconvulsive treatments were often given in a series over several days. Some patients had seven or eight treatments in a row. This therapy was mainly used for depression and schizophrenia.

It was an experience living at the State Psychiatric Hospital in Hastings. The tunnels were really scary, especially the one from the administration building to the nurse's dorm. It was dank, narrow, and dark with only a few lights. It was the home of spiders, cobwebs, and other creatures. I think I used the tunnel once, and that was enough for me! I was glad my assignment was the men's ward. I had the neatest old fellow for my patient. I don't remember his diagnosis anymore, but he was jolly and had a great twinkle in his eyes! He loved to cheat every time we played checkers.

The locked unit was depressing where I saw ECT being administered and the results of ECT on some of the patients. They regressed back to childhood, needing to carry a teddy bear/doll with them. My patient in the locked unit was a young woman, a nurse not much older than myself. That was a difficult assignment. I was really happy to be out of that rotation.

—Judy Mishek Adams

With the advent of the many medications used in treating mental illness since the '60s, electroconvulsive therapy went into decline. It has currently resurfaced and is used primarily for major depression, as well as bipolar disorder and schizophrenia. The patient now has a controlled grand mal seizure during therapy, since muscle relaxants and general anesthesia are administered prior to the procedure.

Psych nursing was like no other that we had previously experienced. Until this time, we had primarily focused on physical aspects in caring for patient needs. We had acquired the many skills of taking care of the bed patient, giving medications, doing treatments and dressing changes, hygiene needs, taking vital signs, observing patient color, breathing, etc. Now, this was different! The patients were ambulatory, and many had behaviors from being institutionalized long term. Some did not want to make eye contact, they paced, some carried many belongings with them, or they spoke inappropriately. As we soon found out.

> "During group therapy, Louie, one of the long-term institutionalized men said, "Take me fishing—Sturgeon Lake?" He had just rolled a cigarette and had tobacco oozing from his mouth as he spoke. His teeth were stained with brown tobacco, and so was his shirt. This comment was totally unrelated to the topic that we were discussing in group. I was trying to think of something to say when he burst out with, "Screwed my wife, didn't I?" I blushed and didn't know what to say! One of the other nurses told him the comment wasn't acceptable in this setting and that he needed to be quiet and pay attention. I really think Louie was incapable of doing that. One never knew what to expect in psych, except to remain composed for whatever might be happening next.
> —Jan Kmieciak Stenson

Besides Thorazine, Stelazine, Compazine, and electroshock therapy, there were few tangible treatments for mental illness. Talk therapy was a tool widely used. Miss Powers and Mrs. Olson, our instructors, both very knowledgeable in dealing with the psych patient, guided us wisely and well. They taught that we must have an awareness of our own feelings in order to be able to focus on our patient. Needless to say, we learned a great deal about our own personalities, and that could sometimes be a bit scary.

Included in talk therapy was a separate entity, group therapy. Patients gathered with the nurses, social worker, and sometimes the physician to discuss different topics. The idea behind this was to provide a safe setting for patients to talk about their feelings, or how to cope with certain situations they might encounter outside of the hospital. In truth, many of the patients had been maintained in the hospital for so many years that they were incapable of functioning in the outside world.

Gradually, we became more comfortable, and we could better understand the psychiatric patient. We were learning how to draw them into a conversation. Developing awareness of nonverbal communication, including body language and eye contact, were skills we hadn't previously been taught. The experience we were having with the psychiatric patient would carry over into dealing with other patients, and into life in general. We were gaining confidence in trusting our instincts in dealing with the patients, but sometimes they really baffled us.

Vicki Lymburner had an incident with Walter one day when she was working on the men's chronic ward. Walter wanted to play shuffleboard with Vicki. With his beaten-down look, he came to ask her to play several times. Finally, she gave in. The shuffleboard court was in the basement of the ward. Vicki and Walter went down the stairs and found the paddles and discs for playing shuffleboard. The game was about to begin when, suddenly, there was Walter face-to-face with Vicki! He pinned her tightly to the equipment rack with his hands pressing on her chest!

Bravely and defiantly, Vicki yelled at Walter, "YOU GET UPSTAIRS RIGHT THIS MINUTE!"

Off Walter scampered to the first floor, and Vicki soon followed in search of our instructor. "I have to talk to you "RIGHT AWAY!" Vicki told the instructor with tears in her eyes. They went into the quiet room, the only private spot. The instructor was able to console Vicki and help her to put the incident in perspective.

Almost fifty years later, we all had a huge chuckle about the incident as only Vicki, in her whimsical style, could tell such a story!

—Jan Kmieciak Stenson

Psych was intriguing for some of us, and others found it difficult to be in this situation. Most everyone loved not having to be under the more rigid rules of Methodist hospital. It felt good to be away, and we had every weekend off, something we hadn't had for a few years. At the dorm we found time to socialize and discuss our patients. We were becoming less concerned with physical assessment of the patient and more adept in using verbal and nonverbal communication. We seemed to be developing more awareness in ourselves, and others. This was a new world.

I had a young woman for my case study while in intensive care. She had schizophrenia, and she had delivered a baby about a month before being admitted to the hospital. She had a "wild" look in her eyes and hardly ever talked. I took her for a walk around the campus, and while walking, she dropped quickly and very hard to her knees! I was shocked by her behavior and didn't know what to do. She was overweight, and I was concerned she had injured her knees. I went back into physical care mode and checked to see if she had injury.

Later, I came to understand that she was most likely hearing voices that were telling her to fall to her knees, and she did, many more times. I asked her what was happening, but I never asked, "Why." Questioning her could have allowed her to become defensive, and there was the possibility her hallucinations might increase.

We were taught to build trust with our patients by being consistent, expecting socially acceptable behavior, and presenting reality whenever we could. Sometimes they told stories that seemed odd and disconnected. We did not tell them that they were wrong. We might say,

"Judy, can you please slow down and tell me one thing at a time. I'm having trouble understanding what you are saying. I've just heard you talk about a school bus, red shoes, and a table."

—Jan Kmieciak Stenson

One day Betty Beard and Vera Kemp arrived at the employee cafeteria for breakfast. Standing outside was a young male patient who was Betty's case study. He visited with them and asked if he could go inside and have breakfast with them. One of them said, "No," and the other said, "Yes." He became enraged and followed them into the cafeteria. At that point, only grape juice and sugar had been set out for breakfast. He began to throw the grape juice and sugar all about the cafeteria! Vera said what she remembers of the incident: "We were very shocked, and the purple color, everywhere, is stuck in my mind!"

After this incident, a meeting was held with Dr. Abuzzahab, the psychiatrist. The nursing students were advised to walk about the campus in pairs.

As part of our coursework, we went to Faribault State Hospital located in Faribault, Minnesota, for a day. It had opened in 1879 to house "idiotic and feeble-minded children." During our visit, we saw very severely and profoundly retarded children, both mentally and physically. Some seemed to be in an almost vegetative state; others were hyperactive. A small girl, perhaps seven or eight years old, with phenylketonuria (PKU) stood and twirled her body back and forth.

This metabolic disorder can be detected with newborn testing and can be successfully treated with diet. There were Downs Syndrome and seizure disorder patients, as well as all types of developmentally disabled children. To see these children, some lying in cribs, others in chairs, some crying pathetically, others constantly moving, was heart wrenching and difficult.

Subsequently, Faribault State Hospital evolved through the years to provide training, treatment, and care in returning persons to live as normal a life as possible within the community. It assisted families in caring for their afflicted family members, fostered public attitudes of understanding and involvement of mental retardation, and conducted research into causes, prevention, and treatment. Faribault State School and Hospital closed in 1998.

During the 1970s, '80s, and '90s, I worked long-term care. Many state hospital patients were admitted after the facilities they had lived in were closing. Edith, a woman in her seventies, told me her sad story one evening. She said she was a young girl of three or four years when one day a social worker came to get her and she was put into an institution. She never saw her mother or family again. Edith seemed mildly developmentally delayed, and it seemed hard to understand why she was taken away. She, certainly, had never understood. Her good friend, Virginia, who also lived at the facility, had uncontrolled seizures and always wore a helmet. She had been institutionalized long term for her seizure disorder. Both women had lived at Faribault State Hospital.

And then there was Gracie. A prefrontal lobotomy had been performed at the state hospital where she had resided. She had a very defiant look on her face as she walked about the home, tightly clutching her purse under her arm. If anyone spoke to her, she usually snapped back with a short phrase, or she totally ignored that person.

A resident in the nursing facility must take a bath once a week for obvious hygiene purposes. Gracie had been requested to take a bath for a few weeks, but she had refused. On this day, her nursing assistant told Gracie that her bathwater was drawn and was waiting for her. She had to take a bath. A while later, the nursing assistant came to get me to ask how to deal with Gracie. I followed her to the tub room. There sat Gracie in the tubful of water, defiantly staring ahead, unwilling to make eye contact. She was fully clothed, wearing her shoes, stockings, coat, and hat, while clutching her purse! She said,"You told me I had to take a bath, so here I am!"

—Carolyn Ukura Kuechle

How different these women's lives might have been had they been born fifty or so years later. Attitudes toward persons with mental and physical afflictions have changed, and families do not feel ashamed as in those days. Antiseizure and antipsychotic medications have become more effective, and psychosurgery, such as prefrontal lobotomies, are considered barbaric and are no longer being performed. Often in our nursing school days, children with special needs had been removed from their family homes and placed in state hospitals because the parents could not financially or emotionally raise them. Education and support services have changed, and now parents have many more resources to tap for assistance. Also, most state hospitals have closed.

However, when budgets are cut, mental health services greatly suffer. While services to clients have changed, we now have people in need of intervention and mental help being housed in prisons, homeless shelters, or worse yet, sleeping on the street. The question remains:

"How do we effectively help people with mental health issues?"

The colors of autumn were beginning to come alive all around us in Hastings. There were many beautiful trees with colorful leaves that were soon falling about the campus. We made our way through crunchy leaves while walking to and from the dorm while on our way to the cafeteria and the hospital wards.

The colorful leaves inspired creativity, and wanting to brighten up the dull gray of the institution, we used them for decorating the walls and the serving table while planning a party for the patients. The party was part of our required curriculum. We were divided into two groups. One group was dressed as turkeys, since it was getting close to Thanksgiving. Our costumes consisted of a burlap bag for the turkey body, beaks made out of surgical masks and orange paper, and turkey feet cut out of orange paper. We did a little dance to the "Turkey Trot." For refreshments, we served punch, cookies, and peanut butter finger sandwiches.

The other group was equally creative, and they came up with a song skit, "Lollipop, Oh, Lollipop," a popular song at the time. The group donned short skirts, knee-high stockings, big hair bows, and held large candy lollipops as props during their "Lollipop, Oh, Lollipop" performance!

On Friday, November 22, 1963, we were looking forward to going home for the weekend. We only had a half-day at the hospital, and there had been no scheduled afternoon class on that memorable day. The sun brightly shone, the skies were a beautiful blue, and it was quite warm for a November day. There seemed to be a peace about the grounds of the hospital.

We had finished our morning on the ward, all had gone well, and soon we would be packing to leave for the weekend. It was lunchtime, and I vividly remember as I was going through the food line in the cafeteria, a patient who worked there on a regular ba-

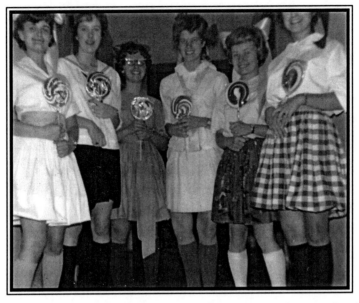

Barb Carlson, Karen Velte, Karen Young, Vera Kemp, Sandy
Morrow, and Vicki Lymburner posing for "Oh, Lollipop!"

sis said to me, "Kennedy was shot."

Of course, I immediately thought this patient
was delusional, and how was I going to present reality
to him while I was getting my food. I said, "Tell me,
how do you know this?"

His reply I assumed was going to be delusional, too, so I was ready.

"On the radio, I just heard it."

Well, I was focused on going home, and he
walked away back to his work. I ate lunch and scampered off to the dorm.

Arriving at the dorm, there was a hush about
the place, the TV was on, and I thought I heard
someone crying. What the heck was going on? One
of my classmates came to tell me that our president
had been shot while riding in an open air car dur-

ing a parade in Dallas, Texas. What the patient in the lunchroom had told me was true. All the TV channels had reporters giving what little information they had about the shooting. We were glued to the TV and we totally forgot about packing. About 1:30 p.m. (Central Standard Time), the news came that our young, vibrant president had died.

What will happen now, I wondered. Surely, whoever did this would be immediately found and put to justice. We all left the hospital quietly, some of us sobbing, and all of us wondering how such a thing could happen. We were stunned, and soon to discover that our parents, friends, and the whole world was stunned as well.

—Jan Kmieciak Stenson

We were experiencing real denial, something we had often discussed in our psych classes. Denial that this could have happened. We heard how Vice President Lyndon Johnson was sworn in as president as his airplane headed back to Washington, DC. He and Lady Bird Johnson had also been riding in the motorcade, a few cars behind President and Jacqueline Kennedy. Days of mourning followed as the president's body lie—first, in the East Room of the White House, then in state in the Capital Rotunda, where there was a constant stream of visitors. President Johnson declared Monday, the twenty-fifth day of November, a national day of mourning, the day of President Kennedy's funeral.

Shockingly, on November 24th, while watching live TV coverage of the aftermath following JFK's assassination, we saw Lee Harvey Oswald, the accused assassin, being escorted from the jail in Dallas, Texas. Out of the crowd stepped a man named Jack Ruby. At close range, he shot Lee Harvey Oswald. Lee Harvey Oswald later died at the same hospital where the president had been taken and pronounced dead.

After this tragic weekend, we were back at Hastings State Hospital on November 25th, and along with the patients in the men's ward, we watched President Kennedy's funeral on TV. This was a very emotional time for everyone, and certainly no less for all the men, even those who were severely emotionally ill. They stood with hands over their hearts at the patriotic songs, and their eyes were riveted to the screen during the entire procession and funeral. We watched the riderless horse, and three-year-old John F. Kennedy, Jr., the president's son, stepping out and standing tall in his short pants and light blue coat to salute his father's flag-draped casket as it was taken out of the cathedral. These were sights that we will never forget.

We went home for the Thanksgiving holiday the Wednesday after President Kennedy's funeral. It was a good time for a break after that very emotional time. In a few more weeks, we would be back to the army-like atmosphere at Methodist Hospital. Psych had brought a new dimension to our nursing knowledge.

Just before Christmas, we departed Hastings State Hospital with new and different skills, and a much greater awareness of the many maladies that can affect the human body and spirit.

Hastings State Hospital closed in 1978. It became the Hastings Veterans Home, as well as a drug rehab center.

CHAPTER 19

Obstetrics and Newborn Nursing

After experiencing psychiatric nursing at Hastings State Hospital, we did a total switch. We began the three-month rotation of obstetrics (OB) and newborns at Methodist Hospital, while those in our class having just experienced OB went to Hastings.

A little more than a month previously, November 22, 1963, the world had experienced the death of President John F. Kennedy. The horrifying events of that day were frozen in memory and would never be forgotten. We personalized and remembered forever where we were on that day. Half of us were on rotation at Hastings State Hospital, and the other half of our class was doing their OB rotation at Methodist Hospital. The effects of that day were in the news then, and continue to this day, fifty years later. President Lyndon B. Johnson's Warren Commission conclusions that Lee Harvey Oswald acted alone in the assassination of President Kennedy have not satisfied the many who believe in conspiracy theories regarding his death. It still is discussed in the media, and books continue to be written about conspiracy theories involving the many players of that time.

President Kennedy's death deeply affected us all, and we had great awareness of it. However, there were other historical 1963 happenings that we hadn't paid as much attention to. The two Cold War superpowers, The United States and the Soviet Union, agreed to establish a "hot line" between the two nations to prevent a possible nuclear war. Martin Luther King, Jr. delivered his "I Have a Dream" speech in Washington, DC, during the March on Washington for jobs and freedom that helped spawn the 1964 Civil Rights Act. The United States was getting deeper into the Vietnam War in 1963 that turned into a long and costly war and divided the nation.

Changes were on the horizon for women and families in the United States with Betty Friedan's book, *The Feminine Mystique*. It was published in 1963. In her role as a housewife, scrubbing and waxing her linoleum floor to perfection, Betty Friedan asked: "Is this all?"

Millions of women across the country began to ask the same question after reading *The Feminine Mystique*. From this writing, the women's movement began.

Studying hard, working, and trying our best to get through the rigors of nursing school in 1963 didn't allow much time to read *The Feminine Mystique*. However, it wasn't long before we acquired awareness of the struggles inherent in the women's movement. In the end, that movement affected us all.

In the dorm at Methodist Hospital, we knew of The Beatles, a rock band from Liverpool, England. They began releasing their music in 1963 and appeared on the *Ed Sullivan Show* in early 1964. The four young men, John Lennon, Paul McCartney, George Harrison, and Ringo Starr, wrote their own music and had a definite style. They became wildly popular, and the description of them, their music, and their popularity was coined "Beatlemania."

We were given an orientation to third floor, where the entire floor of the hospital was devoted to maternity care. There were six labor rooms, three delivery rooms, and capacity for six separate nurseries, one being a pre-term nursery. Fifty to fifty-five maternity patients could be accommodated at a time.

Mrs. Terhaar, whom we had as our surgical instructor, was also the OB instructor. She had had much obstetrical experience. She was a graduate of Mercy School of Nursing in Iowa. Not only was she with us during our clinical experience, she also taught the classroom theory portion in her monotonous "twang." There was a certain dread in having her as the primary instructor, since she could be quite ornery and tended not to sugar coat anything. Not that we expected her to, but we would have preferred a kinder approach. We wondered how the patients perceived her with her black unkempt hair, wire rimmed glasses, old-fashioned long sleeved, yellowish white uniforms, and sharply pointed nurse's cap. Her old-fashioned shoes made a clopping sound, so we knew when she was nearby. She seemed to have come from the dark ages.

We learned about the female body inside and out. If only I had known then that I would one day be in Mrs. Terhaar's place teaching OB in Iowa, I would have paid better attention to what I was learning!
—Jan Kmieciak Stenson

Our OB experience included observing and caring for women in the labor, delivery, and postpartum rooms, while learning the needed skills to do so. And then it was onto the newborn and preterm infant nurseries. We worked with very experienced nurses who were willing and helpful in teaching student nurses.

Soon-to-be moms, arriving at the hospital in various stages of labor, were directed to a labor room, and the admitting process was begun. An abdominal examination was performed to determine size, position, and presentation of the fetus, as well as noting the presence of fetal heart tones. An estimate of the quality, duration, and frequency of contractions was noted. A vaginal exam was performed to determine dilation of the cervix to allow passage of the fetus. Dilatation of the cervix was measured in centimeters from zero to ten. Ten centimeters was indicative of imminent delivery of the child.

Generally, a labor of twelve to fourteen hours is common for a woman who had not previously delivered a child, but much shorter for a woman who had had multiple births. In the latter situation, the labor time could go very quickly! The experienced nurses were aware and ready for all possibilities in birthing, from a very long and tedious labor to a quick "Now we are at ten!" This situation would require a fast trip down the hall into the delivery room!

Distress to the fetus during the birthing process could be indicated by the fetal heart rate. Therefore, the rate was closely monitored for changes in rate and intensity. Fetal heart tones were taken every fifteen minutes during early labor. As the contractions of labor progressed, they were taken after every contraction. A stethoscope attached to a metal band that slipped over the nurse or MD's head was used in listening for fetal heart tones.

I was on night duty with a mother-to-be during labor. I went into her room with a headband stethoscope to check the fetal heart beat. I was wearing contact lenses in my eyes (the hard style). As I put on the headband and leaned over the mother's abdomen to listen for the fetal heart tone, the headband pulled back, and out of my eye popped my contact! Down it went into the bed with the large, laboring, uncomfortable mom. Talk about a foolishly feeling, flustered student nurse trying to explain this silly incident to my patient. Luckily, we both could laugh! I moved her about in the bed and finally found the lens. I got it back into my eye so I could see again and got back to work.
—Karen Young Miller

In addition to monitoring fetal heart tones, there was constant monitoring of the cervix during labor. There was a contraption called the "Birth Ease" in use at that time for easing the mom's discomfort during contractions. This was a large plastic dome that was placed over the uterus and attached to some sort of air pressure device. We all had the opportunity to try the device. It was a feeling of suction that we experienced over our abdomen. There were few drugs administrated during labor. A type of spinal block, known as the "saddle block," was occasionally given. This numbed the region of the body that would sit on a saddle.

> Back in those days, they used this suction dome on the abdomen. The laboring patient pushed a button that would help to lift the abdomen to supposedly help to relieve some of the pain from the contraction. Personally, I don't think it helped. That technique didn't last long.
> —Judy Mishek Adams

The laboring patient was wheeled into the delivery room when her cervix dilatation was at or near ten centimeters, or she was verbalizing the need to push down with contractions. We felt it was quite a privilege to be observing the birthing of a baby as we accompanied a soon-to-be mom to the delivery room.

During class time, we were shown films on babies being birthed. This was exciting, but to see the real thing was amazing! We were on call to go to the labor and delivery to see a birth. We saw how the mothers used all their strength to bear down and push the baby into the world. We heard the baby's cry and saw the mother's joy and relief! She saw the miracle she had created after nine months of carrying this growing child in her body. The discomforts she had encountered during pregnancy, labor, and delivery now appeared to be forgotten.

After delivery of the baby, its mouth cleaned with a bulb syringe, and it had begun crying and breathing, the umbilical cord was cut. A general delivery room inspection of the baby was made, including the Apgar scoring. This system rated an infant's physical condition at one minute and five minutes after birth. Wrapped in a blanket, the baby was given to the mother to hold and check over. A 1 percent silver nitrate solution was instilled in each of the infant's eyes. This was given as a blindness preventative from gonorrheal infection that might be present in the mother's birth canal. A nurse from the newborn nursery came to take the baby from the delivery room after a matching identification bracelet to the mother was placed on the baby. A primary concern after birth was that the baby's temperature be maintained.

After the placenta had been expelled from the uterus, the new mom was taken from the delivery room to a postpartum room. Her vital signs were closely monitored. We were instructed in how to find the fundus of the uterus, located one to two centimeters below the umbilicus. It should be firm, if not, it could indicate bleeding. Something as simple as a full bladder might interfere with firming. A gentle massage of the fundus to help the uterus to contract was shown us, and we practiced this skill. The lochia discharge from the uterus was closely observed for amount and color.

> I was amazed to find the fundus while caring
> for a newly delivered patient, and we, later, learned
> in class about the efficiency of the uterus both in ex-
> panding and contracting.
> —Jan Kmieciak Stenson

Caring for postpartum (directly after birth) women was usually a fun experience! They normally were in a happy frame of mind, and they didn't need a lot of hands-on care. They were up and about, and they could shower on their own, unless they'd had a Cesarean birth (C-section). The new mothers normally had a hospital stay of four to five days in 1963–64. They relaxed and spent time with their baby, who was brought to them from the nursery, and returned to the nursery. And, they attended classes on baby care.

> We were on a three-month rotation in OB, and as we gained proficiency, we had our first experience with actually teaching patients. We did infant bath demonstrations and helped the moms with infant care, including bottle and breast-feeding. Most of the infants were fed on demand; they cried and were fed, usually quieting them. I often wondered what the mothers were thinking when a young woman was teaching them about something the experienced mothers most likely already knew.
> —Jan Kmieciak Stenson

The La Leche (Spanish for "the milk") League visited the OB department at Methodist hospital to educate, encourage, and help willing new mothers get started in breast-feeding. Formula bottle-feeding (around 80 percent) was the preferred method for feeding babies at that time. The La Leche League promoted breast milk as the superior and natural infant food that it is and promoted bonding between mother and child. In the United States today, more babies are breastfed than bottle fed.

Newborn Nursery
After stabilization of temperature, the newborn was weighed and measured, given a bath, dressed, and swaddled tightly in a blanket. The child was closely observed for color, breathing, vomiting, ability to urinate, sucking and rooting reflexes, and passing of stools, noting color and amount. The normal newborn could be fed immediately after birth. A complete physical exam by the physician was performed within the first twelve hours of birth.

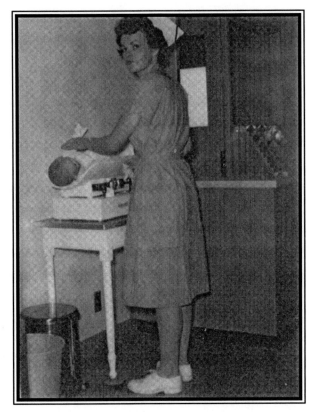

Velma Jean Shelton weighing baby.

At first we merely observed in the newborn nursery, but soon we were able to care for the babies. It was a fun place to be as we bathed, diapered, dressed, and sometimes fed the infants. The baby was wheeled in its isolette to the mother's room, always matching mother to baby armbands. To watch the new mom with her baby was a delight! When the mother called, we returned the baby to the nursery. Generally today, babies are kept with the mother in the same private room.

Preterm Infant Nursery
Premature infants are those born before thirty-seven weeks gestation. These infants have a more difficult time getting started in the

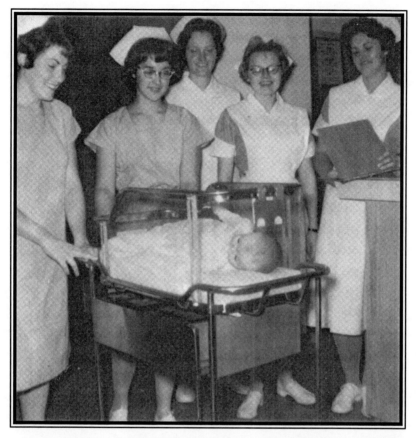

Learning about newborns: Judy March, Sandy Johnson, Beth
Johnson, Judy Stoneback, and Judy Mishek.

world, but most catch up with time. They offer many more challenges
in caring for them than normal newborns, and many opportunities in
learning.

The premies were placed in the preterm nursery, where they
received close monitoring and specialized care. Airway and breathing
were the first conditions to be addressed, since the infant's lungs were
not adequately developed. Sucking and swallowing reflexes weren't
coordinated well enough yet to allow normal eating. Temperature
regulation was another issue, since they could quickly lose body heat.
Preventing infection required closely adhered to infection control

procedures. The premies appeared very fragile with no fat and very thin skin through which their blood vessels could be seen. It took courage to work with them for fear of harming them. Fortunately, we had a confident, knowledgeable head nurse who was able to impart her confidence to us. She demonstrated how to do a gavage feeding with a tiny premie, and made it appear easy.

Being in the nursery, I found it fun to take care of newborns. The preterm nursery, however, was quite different. The premies, often, were very tiny; some weighed less than two pounds. At that time, retrolental fibroplasia, a disease of the retina of the eye that could cause blindness, was just beginning to be understood. The disorder was associated with too high a concentration of administered oxygen.

We soon learned just how to handle these tiny infants by using the palm of our hand placed on the infant's chest to turn its small body. We were closely instructed in giving a premie a gavage feeding. The procedure was similar to working with an adult to place a tube into the stomach. After the tube was placed, a syringe was attached to the tube opening. Formula was poured into the syringe and allowed to run into the stomach by gravity. When possible, the premie was fed by gavage for one feeding, while the next feeding was a bottle feeding. Due to its weak sucking reflex, it took a lot of the tiny baby's energy to suck even 5cc (one teaspoon) of formula. This was a complicated procedure with a tiny, fragile patient. Though I wasn't, I felt very skilled after accomplishing it.

—Jan Kmeiciak Stenson

There were, of course, complicated pregnancies, and not all deliveries proceeded normally. If a fetus began to indicate it was in distress during labor, or a cervix did not dilate, or for other reasons, an emergency C-section was performed. After a C-section was performed, any subsequent pregnancies ended up as C-sections. And, of course, there were planned C-sections. Postpartum care for a mom who had had a C-section included surgical nursing care, as well.

Perhaps the saddest situation during our OB rotation was a baby delivered who had anencephalus. This child had an absence of brain, skull, and scalp. It never gained consciousness, and died the day after birth. This is a very rare occurrence.

In today's world, many changes and advances have occurred in obstetrics. New moms only stay in the hospital a day or two after delivery. Prenatal care includes ultrasounds that show how things are going in the uterus, including determining the gender of the fetus or if there might be multiple fetuses. There are fewer surprises at delivery. Amniocentesis, a needle biopsy of amniotic fluid, is more refined to allow studies of the amniotic fluid to detect genetic or biochemical disorders, if deemed necessary. There no longer is a one size fits all in birthing. Hospitals have improved their maternity wards to offer more options than just lying in a bed during labor. Women can choose natural childbirth or have an epidural (spinal anesthetic) or other measures for pain. Fathers, and sometimes others, are allowed to be in the delivery room.

There is more family orientation with siblings allowed to visit mom and the new baby. Babies remain in the room with the mother most of the time. Now, there are midwives who deliver babies, and doulas who work and support a pregnant woman during pregnancy, labor, and delivery, and after the birth. Lactation consultants work with breast-feeding mothers, and there are electric breast pumps, a tool that encourages moms to breast-feed. There are education classes offered to couples; thus, fathers have become far more involved in the birthing process and are able to better support the mom during labor. They are more involved in their children's care, as well. A win-win for all!

The one thing that stands out in my memory during our OB rotation was the November 1963 assassination of President John F. Kennedy while riding in a motorcade in Dallas, Texas. Everyone was totally stunned—unbelievable! Classes were cancelled that afternoon.

When we had our preterm nursery rotation, it was a really super experience working with isolettes, gavage feeding the premies, and just taking care of them. Some weighed not much more than a pound. This experience helped me tremendously after graduation when I worked OB and preterm nursery. Occasionally, it was necessary for me to teach a four-year grad how to do a gavage feeding, as she had not had that opportunity during her nursing school education.
—Judy Mishek Adams

We encountered a very large change about halfway through our obstetrics rotation.

I remember being in clinical in the labor unit. There wasn't much going on, so we were going through cabinets and learning about instruments. Others in the class were in the nursery and postpartum areas. It was a Friday, and we had finished our clinical hours for the week. We reported off the unit and went to lunch. After lunch, most of us went back to the dorm to put our feet up, relax, smoke, make phone calls, watch TV, or just gab.

At 1:30 p.m., we reported for class in one of the nursing school classrooms. There was an "eerie" feeling about the area when we arrived. We were told that Mrs. Terhaar, from whom we were to have class, had become ill. She had had a heart attack, and very suddenly, Mrs. Terhaar had died. Few details were given, but apparently, other instructors in the area had administered CPR to no avail.

Of course, we all were very shocked! We were told to study on our own until further notice. No doubt Mrs. Terhaar's death was causing shock and turmoil to Miss Barber and the instructors in the nursing school, as well. They now had three levels of classes to teach, and an instructor knowledgeable in OB was needed. We dreamed up all sorts of scenarios as to what would happen during the remainder of our rotation. Most of us dutifully went to the funeral home to pay our respects to Mrs. Terhaar, who had tried her best to teach us. While we realized we hadn't always appreciated her intensity and straight forwardness, we felt sad at her passing, as she had given us much hands-on and useful knowledge.

We had concerns that we would not know OB well enough to pass the Minnesota State Board exam in July. To Miss Barber's tribute, on Monday we were told that a nurse from the hospital, studying to be a nurse midwife, a very new area in nursing, would become our instructor. Most of us had gotten to know her from clinical and had found her to be very helpful and knowledgeable. She was a good choice.

—Jan Kmieciak Stenson

Again, it was a change, but we found our new instructor added another dimension to our knowledge of obstetrics with her very practical experience and teaching ability. We adapted. We seemed to be getting good at that. We looked forward to the final rotation, pediatrics. And soon, graduation!

CHAPTER 20

Pediatric Nursing

It was March of 1964, and we were heading into the homestretch of our three years of nursing school. Care of children was our last three-month rotation. The pediatrics (peds) unit was located on fourth floor at Methodist Hospital, where there was capacity for forty-six children in double rooms and pediatric wards. The children were grouped by age and diagnosis.

Winter was beginning to turn into longer, spring-like days with warmer temps. We knew, along with the more pleasant weather, that studying was going to become more difficult. Another factor, of course, was that we were nearing the end and reaching saturation for being in school. We were looking forward to our first real nurse job! Two classmates had married, and several more were engaged.

Our challenge now was to learn nursing care of sick kids. We began by learning about the growth and development of the normal infant and child before learning about the diseases of the infant, toddler, preschooler, school-age child, and adolescent. This included expected milestones of each age group, such as walking, talking, dressing and undressing without assistance, learning colors, etc. We learned about immunizations, nutrition, generalized behavioral, and intellectual development from infant to adolescent.

Miss Dorothy Dobratz was our pediatrics instructor. She had a relaxed demeanor, a hearty laugh, and didn't seem stiff or stressed.

She related well to children of all ages, as well as to student nurses. Sometimes she came to the dorm and watched soap operas or played cards. Further, she knew pediatrics well, and she displayed common sense. We affectionately referred to her as "Dobie."

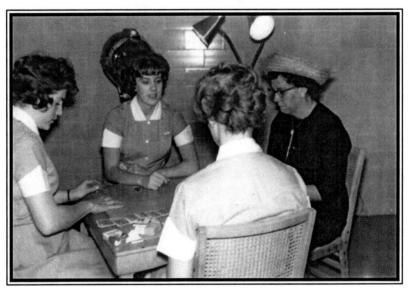

Miss Dobratz, on the left, playing cards at the dorm.

I had observed Miss Dobratz while working for pay on the weekends. I thought her to be in her thirties. As a child, she had polio and walked with a limp, but she got around very well. She was cheery, laughed a lot, and told jokes. She'd had extensive pediatric experience and was a graduate of Abbott Hospital School of Nursing in Minneapolis.

I had been working on the peds unit for two and a half years by this time. I had observed many pediatric nurse styles of communication with the children. Some I would never emulate, but being low on the totem pole, I said little. Miss Dobratz had a reassuring and caring style of communication, and she inspired this in her teaching. We were "antsy" to move on, and Dobie probably sensed that. Her easy-going style was a gift.

The first day of theory class, Miss Dobratz talked about occupations. *Occupations? Really, how does this relate to pediatrics?* I wondered.

She asked, "What is the occupation of a seven year old child?"

We all looked at each other, and no one raised a hand or made eye contact with Dobie. Then she told us the child's occupation is play. I thought, *Well, that was a really easy question.* I hadn't realized how elementary and true it was!

—Jan Kmieciak Stenson

There were illnesses related to the season of the year. Upper respiratory, pneumonia, and croup were seen in winter, and with spring came vomiting and diarrhea (V and D). Most respiratory conditions were treated with antibiotics and the child was placed in a humidity room.

Vomiting and diarrhea was most common in infants and toddlers. It usually was inflammation of the stomach and/or intestine caused by a bacterial or viral organism. The child was miserable, cried, filled its diaper, and wouldn't eat or drink. It was very challenging to get the child to drink fluids to maintain hydration. The offending organism usually "ran its course" and the child returned to health in a few days.

Keeping an IV going in children was a major concern. The younger the child, the more they wriggled and moved, and the less likely an IV could work.

A child with diarrhea was usually placed in isolation to lessen contagion to others. Isolation technique included good hand washing practice and wearing a gown whenever caring for the child. Dirty laundry and wastes had to be double bagged and placed in isolation areas. Sometimes nurses caught the "diarrhea bug." Miss Dobratz knew that hand washing had not been adequate when that happened.

It was a very busy pediatrics unit at Methodist with children having surgery, the wet rooms with humidity for croup and asthma patients, and the isolation wards. I remember Miss Dobratz saying when working the isolation rooms, "If you get sick, you didn't wash your hands well, and you didn't follow isolation technique." (Anyway, something to that effect.)

The worst experience I had in peds was having my patient be a three-year-old child, whom I had babysat, and having to give her a penicillin shot. I was never asked to babysit for that family again. Most likely because the parents thought the little girl would identify me with the shot, and she would be afraid of me. My work for pay experience was in peds. Apparently, it was my best subject, since I received my highest State Board of Nursing score in it. A few years after graduation, I worked in a peds unit in a small community hospital, taking care of very sick children who had both serious medical and surgical problems. My previous education and experience at Methodist was very helpful.

—Judy Mishek Adams

Pediatric medications were more challenging, both in figuring dosages for accuracy and while administrating. We learned to give all age groups injectable antibiotics, such as penicillin, Declomycin, and Chloromycetin. A tubex syringe held a premeasured penicillin dose that had to be placed into the metal holder for administration. This was more awkward than using a normal syringe. To readily get the injection done, cause the least trauma, and offer the child reassurance, we always had a helper.

Used hypodermic needles are never recapped in this era of HIV/AIDS. In those days before HIV/AIDS had reared its ugly head, needles were always recapped. Sometimes a nurse would stick herself with the used needle. Blood and body fluids were merely washed off and forgotten.

> Since many times we were required to determine a dosage from the medication label, Miss Dobratz taught the basic algebraic equation to figure "x." She quizzed us in both class and clinical to be sure we could do the math. At first it seemed a daunting task, but then it became quite easy. The equation became like second nature, and one had to master it to work in peds. Little did I know that one day I'd be teaching this to my own students.
> —Jan Kmieciak Stenson

Children having surgery were admitted to the pediatric unit the evening before their procedure. The parents did not stay the night with the child, but returned the next day. The child was admitted around 6:00 p.m., was introduced to the unit, saw the playroom, and had a light supper. Visiting hours were over at 7:30 p.m. The parents went home, and the child was bedded down for the night. This worked for the older children who settled down and went to sleep. Toddlers and preschoolers cried and needed much attention without their parents nearby.

The next day, the child was pulled in a little red wagon to the operating room. The child's parents trailed along behind. Once in the surgical area, the parents went to the waiting room while their child was taken into surgery. Most of the children who had elective surgeries, such as tonsil and adenoid removal, hernias, and myringotomies (incision of the ear drum for relief of infection), came to a presurgical tour a week prior to surgery. This helped to decrease anxiety for the child and parents.

Tonsil and adenoid removal (T and As) were frequently done then; now it is less common. The child was usually given ether for an anesthetic, and the ether fumes lingered after surgery return. Some of us had watched the T and A procedure during our surgery rotation. It was a bloody procedure, and when the child coughed up blood post-op, it didn't seem like such a "big deal." Many of the children had nausea and vomiting (N and V) related to the ether. They did not want to eat or drink, but often they would eat ice cream and popsicles. Children seemed more resilient than adults after surgery. They were often up and walking about by afternoon, and they were discharged the following morning. Currently, this procedure is done on an out-patient basis.

In the '60s, there were no rules in place regarding length of hospital stay or insurance dictates regarding payment.

On the peds unit, there were children with broken bones, in-cluding arms, fingers, legs, and occasionally, a skull fracture. A child with a fractured femur (thigh bone) would be placed in traction for four to six weeks to keep the bone in proper alignment, or have a "hip-spica" cast applied to the trunk of the body and leg. Sometimes, sur-gery was necessary, but it wasn't the norm. There were many nursing challenges in maintaining a child's position to promote proper heal-ing and very close monitoring to prevent skin irritation. The immobi-lized child was not a happy child. Oftentimes, the child experienced pain and was irritable. In these situations, play therapy was important.

Part of our peds rotation involved being the "play lady" for a week. The week in clinical as play lady was to go about the unit and find appropriate toys for the children to engage them in play. This was a distraction from the tediousness of being a hospital patient, helped relieve them of boredom while being immobilized, and moved the time along while they were healing. It was a good learning opportunity for us. We did a project for a specific age group and presented it in class. Later, we found there were state board exam questions on this very subject.

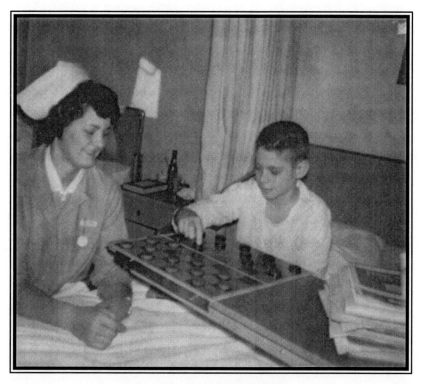

Judy Mishek as the play lady.

Methodist Hospital had several pediatricians on staff. Dr. Etzweiler specialized in endocrine disorders of children, and he came to speak on juvenile-onset diabetes. At this time, he was doing research on how well newly graduated nurses understood diabetes, and he welcomed this teaching opportunity. Type II diabetes had been included in our previous med-surg unit and was referred to as adult-onset diabetes. The pancreas may produce insulin, but over time, the cells become resistant to it. There were oral medications coming on the market for treatment of adult-onset diabetes in the '60s. Fortunately, today there are many highly effective oral medications.

Type I, or juvenile-onset diabetes, is a different situation. Due to absolute insulin deficiency, juvenile-onset diabetes was treated only with insulin injection, as it still is today.In general, all nurses will encounter patients with diabetes in any setting, and they must have a good working knowledge of this disorder. The good Doctor Etzweiler had a way of explaining this fascinating, but complex, disease so we would understand it well.

Urine diabetic testing is no longer routinely done. Now, using a meter, a person with diabetes will collect a drop or two of blood and get an accurate readout of their blood sugar. Fortunately, there have been many advances made in both Type I and Type II diabetes mellitus treatment. There are more effective oral medications, insulin pumps, education in prevention of Type II diabetes, and how to live a healthy lifestyle with diabetes.

Today there are nurses who specialize in diabetes management. They teach people with diabetes how to administer medication, when and how to self-test for blood sugar levels, educate awareness in symptoms of low or high blood sugar, balance diet with exercise, and offer support for what is a lifetime endeavor. Unfortunately, with higher rates of obesity in children, Type II diabetes is being diagnosed in children of today's world.

We also saw congenital disorders in peds. I remember holding a little boy with dark, rather long hair, and large for his age. His legs, arms, and head were about the size of a two year old, and he was quite heavy. He couldn't hold up his head well, and he drank from a nipple and bottle. The pediatrician suspected that this child had a form of giantism, a rare condition. We saw kids with clubfeet (feet turned inward), Down's syndrome, hip dysplasia (congenital bone malformation resulting in hip dislocating), and hydrocephalus (increased cerebrospinal fluid in the

brain). Some of these conditions could be treated, while others had little treatment possibilities. A child with hydrocephalus had frequent "taps"(drainage of cerebrospinal fluid), to decrease pressure in the brain.
—Jan Kmieciak Stenson

We had the usual obligatory case study, as we had had in all other specialty areas. This involved researching the subject, finding photos, if possible, writing, or typing the final draft if we had typewriter access. We had many speakers during class time. Some were very good; others we didn't feel did as well. And, of course, we were tested at least once a week.

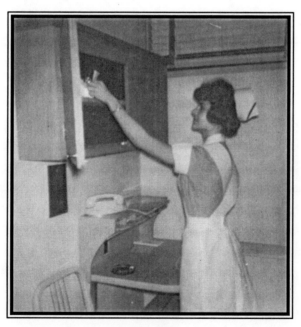

Sue Tingerthal visiting the Saint Louis Park Clinic while on pediatric rotation.

We also had a special case study that involved teaching a child about their disease process. The child had to be school age or older to comprehend our educational challenge! I found myself trying to teach a ten year old how his kidneys worked. He had been diagnosed with acute glomerulonephritis. This disease was rather common on our unit, and it may be caused by certain strains of streptococci after respiratory infection. It caused swelling, irritability, and weight gain. The treatment was to keep the child at rest, give a special low-salt diet to help decrease edema (swelling), and obtain frequent urine tests to assess kidney function.

I had come up with the idea of using a strainer as a way to explain what the kidney did. I found pictures for the child to understand his disease. I made projects for him to color or cut out, as these would keep him at rest. I honestly never really knew if he understood a word that I was telling him.

—Jan Kmieciak Stenson

Pediatrics was quite a rewarding experience, partly because it was our last rotation, and we were near the end, but also because we felt we had learned a lot. We had gained a level of comfort in knowing how to impart information to children, and their parents. We had learned some common sense methods, such as putting pills into jelly to get the kids to take them. Soon we would be out in the working world, testing what we thought we knew against what was expected of us. No longer would there be an instructor to fall back upon. Each of us would be on her own.

Of course, we all were focusing on the culmination of our three years of nursing education and experience, the taking of Minnesota State Board of Nursing examination. Only after passing all five parts of the test would we become registered nurses.

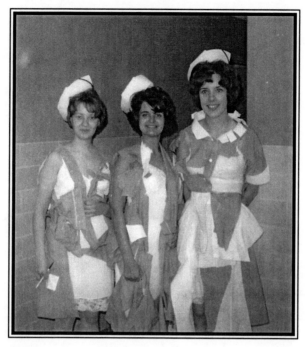

The last day, wearing no-longer-needed, torn-into-rags student
uniforms! Carolyn Ukura, Barbara Carlson, and Karen Velte.

CHAPTER 21

Love Stories

Blind Date Turns to Marriage

A I am twenty years old, and in my senior year at Methodist Hospital School of Nursing.

One evening, my cousin, who lived in Saint Paul, phoned to ask if I might be interested in meeting a very nice young man whom she had met in a summer school class at the University of Minnesota. He had struck up a conversation with her. She, being the friendly type, had made him think that she might be interested in him. He asked her out more than once; however, each time she told him she was already pinned and in a serious relationship. Finally, she told him she had a cousin who was going to nursing school in Saint Louis Park, and she may be interested in going with him on a blind date. Thus, my cousin phoned me.

I had gone on a few blind dates before, and they hadn't been very successful. I was dating someone, but not seriously. I mulled it over for a few days and realized that this would be a totally blind date. We would be meeting with only each other. Typically, a blind date meant you were with another couple who had set you up. I admired my cousin, and knew we had similar values, so I didn't think she would set me up with a loser! The next time that I talked to my cousin, I told her to give him my phone number.

A few days later, he called me. We set up a date to go to The Old Log Theater to see a play, and then to go out for pizza.

The following is an excerpt from my husband, Lee Clift, in the journal that he wrote twenty years later, when he was dying of cancer.

We met through a blind date arranged by cousin Norene. I expected a blond Scandinavian about five foot, six inches. The last Johnson I had met at the U was very attractive and fit that description. So, of course, Sandy would be just like that. Sandy was also supposed to be wearing a black plaid coat. It was a cool weekend in late October 1963.

Sandy's blond hair was a little dark, and her plaid coat was a check, but her smile

was just what I had hoped for, and expected, of a Johnson, and a cousin of Norene.

I had enrolled in summer school for one purpose: to meet a nice girl. After several attempts to arrange a date with Norene, I was convinced she would remain true to her future husband, Larry. I was sure glad she did not hang up on me before telling me about her cousin.

We went to the Old Log Theater, and then for pizza in Saint Louis Park. We both remember being concerned about eating pizza with long, stringy cheese.

Sandy doesn't count our quick kiss at the door as being our first. She remembers the second, which we had to practice a couple of times.

After our first date, I predicted that I would marry, "that girl," to a fellow teacher.

Deer hunting interfered with the next Saturday night, but we managed coffee at Mr. Q's restaurant, the night President John F. Kennedy was assassinated.

Another weekend, I remember, we went to a play at the Orpheum, and not wanting to appear too stingy, I got the second least expensive tickets. This got us into the second to the last row!

We visited her folks and family at the farm for a weekend in early December, and discovered the perils of glare ice, and snowstorm, on a roller skate— it was my 1962 VW.

I met the whole clan on Christmas Eve as Santa came rolling in (somersaulting Uncle Wally). Sandy has a very large family, and I memorized many names that night.

We went skiing with many friends on January 6, 1964. We had a great time. We've skied once a year since. Sandy asked me what I had in mind for our future at a movie that evening. Although I have never admitted it, I probably would have pursued the subject myself, if she hadn't brought it up then. Aha! I got you!

We did see the movie *Irma La Douce*, (a romantic comedy with Jack Lemmon and Shirley McLaine) when we first started dating. Did that movie influence our romantic style for years to come?

We stuck to the traditional. I asked her dad for his daughter's hand in marriage as we were going to witness her roommate, and future husband's, elopement. It was difficult for Dad to say, "No," to a kid with a sparkly new ring in his lapel pocket. He did wonder why we didn't wait a while, but somehow we got by that, and I gave her the ring that night!

I thought to myself, how many of the rest of
the marriages started with that bit of tradition intact?

We were married in October 1964 at a small town church. I cherish these words that he wrote about our blind date and courtship. When he died, we had been married twenty-one and a half years, and we had three wonderful sons.

What happens in one's life is never predictable, but the human spirit continues in hope, and has the capacity to express love in new ways that continue to enrich life.
—Sandy Johnson Clift Ware

Checking the Time Cards

As a student nurse, you could almost always have a date if you wanted one. Somehow, the word got out to fraternity groups, and others, that nurses were available. There were coffee dates, dinner and movie dates, or just going for a walk. Some of us went to see the musical, *West Side Story*, three or four times. The music was fantastic. And then there was *Cape Fear*, a real thriller. The poignant *Days of Wine and Roses* showed us Jack Lemmon portraying an alcoholic. Of course, it wasn't long before the James Bond series captured us. Remember *Goldfinger*? And, who could forget the Alfred Hitchcock excitement in *The Birds*. In the '60s, seeing a movie cost about eighty-five cents to two dollars. Dinner averaged somewhere around $3.75. I do remember movies being the most popular thing to do on a date, rather than going to dinner.

It was June 1962, and I was back home, but working full-time at Methodist Hospital. Sometimes, my dad or brother would drive me to the hospital for that early 7:00 a.m. start. One morning on our way to the hospital, we noticed a young man biking along the road. My dad assumed this guy was going to work, and he thought it was good that he was using muscle power to get around. Being quite naïve, and disinterested, I didn't make any comment.

Most of us had lots of dates during the school year. There were orderlies, guys from hometowns, blind dates, and some doctors wanting to date student nurses. Some of the class had boyfriends, and they were looking for dates for their friends. Word seemed to spread that student nurses were "fun" to date.

I remember right after I had cleaned out my room for the summer, I saw new faces near the time clock. Two guys, one short, one tall, and near my age, strode onto the elevator one day.

I began to see these guys in the cafeteria and while they were on their way to housekeeping. At that time, I was working in pediatrics on the fourth floor. We often had children diagnosed with meningitis, and their rooms were "fogged" as part of the cleaning process after discharge. A fogging machine, like those used for backyard mosquitoes, was used in any room in the hospital that had had an infectious disease. An antibacterial solution was mixed and poured into the fogger. The housekeeping department was responsible for this cleaning, so the "newcomer" guys donned gown, gloves, cap, and mask to fog the room. All the furniture in the room was wiped clean. This was a time-consuming process that often had to be done within the pediatric unit.

One day, the tall guy came into the peds unit and was fogging a room. I didn't think too much of it, and I went about my work checking temperatures, feeding toddlers, giving baths, and cleaning cabinets. At the end of the day, I saw this fellow without his mask as I was leaving the unit. I walked by, and I casually said, "Hi." He looked at me, but he didn't say a word. I didn't think anything of it and went about my way down to the time clock.

The next morning I saw these two new workers at the time clock again. So, I just hustled off to work. I noticed these guys around the hospital. Then one day, the tall one said, "Hi." *How about that*, I thought, *he does have a voice.*

About a week later, I was at home with my parents and siblings watching *The Munsters* on TV. The phone rang. I answered and found myself talking to Chuck, the tall guy from the hospital. I thought he must be calling to know someone's name, since there were several of us working at the hospital. Wrong! He asked me for a date. I hardly remembered what he had said, and I didn't get his last name right.

Little did I know that Chuck would be my future husband. We were both nineteen, and each of us had completed one year of college. We began dating, and sometimes we double-dated with another classmate, Monyne, and her future husband, Fred. Soon, he was picking me up and dropping me off from work.

Too soon, summer was over, and it was back to the books for both of us. Chuck went back to college in Iowa, and I returned to Methodist. Later that year, Chuck told me he had gone through all the time cards one day to get the spelling of my name so he could call me for a date!

—Jan Kmieciak Stenson

Karen and Brad's Crazy Love Story

I was in my second year of nursing school. I was looking forward to a weekend off from work, and I was planning to drive home to Alden. Have '53 Chevy, will travel.

I received a phone call from Toni, who lived in the neighboring town of Freeborn. She was attending the Minnesota School of Business in Minneapolis. She wanted to know if she and her boyfriend, Brad, could get a ride home with me. I told her I would pick them up on Friday afternoon.

Jane Fulton, my friend from Alden, was a first-year student at Methodist Hospital School of Nursing, and she was also going to ride home with me. On Friday afternoon, Jane and I set out to pick up Brad and Toni, and the four of us headed south to Freeborn/Alden. The trip was uneventful, and we had safe travels home.

I was to leave Brad and Toni off at his parents' home, a mile or so outside of Freeborn. And, I did. I pulled into the driveway. I got out of the Chevy to open the trunk for their luggage. Brad took the luggage and handed me a ten-dollar bill. I took the money, said "Thanks," jumped back into the car, and took off down the road. As I drove off, he said he stood there with his mouth open and hand out. He was waiting and thinking I would give him some change for his ten dollars. I guess it was an expensive trip home for the farm boy.

About a year later, I took some of my nursing classmates home to Alden, and we went dancing to "The Bubble." There I met up with Brad once again. We started dating that led to courtship, and wedding bells rang out in April 1965. Then it was life on the farm, two great children, and five beautiful grandchildren. I guess it all turned out—the money is ours!

One last note: Brad always said, "I had to marry her to get my money back!"

—Karen Young Miller

CHAPTER 22

A Different Course Ahead: The Novice

By: Jan Kmieciak Stenson

It was May 1964. Our nursing school days were coming to an end, and reality was setting in. We had completed all the necessary classes in specialty areas, and what remained were four weeks of classes in disaster nursing, legal aspects, nurse management, and leadership. There were a few paperback books to read, but no papers to write or projects to present in our classwork. We had one day a week of classroom and four entire days working on the hospital units.

In the disaster nursing course, we read and discussed the paperback book, *Hiroshima*. It told of the ravages of atomic warfare and its aftermath. We studied the horrible effects of burns and radiation poisoning from atomic bombs. Our country was getting deeper and deeper into the "Cold War," and there was awareness that the wrong button could be pushed to launch the delivery of atom bombs with serious casualties. Being prepared and informed, and knowing what we could do in a disaster to help people and possibly save lives, was the gist of the course. The magnitude of such a situation could hardly be comprehended. Further, since we hadn't had much time to pay attention to the world's problems, an atomic attack seemed mostly like fiction. We were in our own learning world.

Legal aspects of nursing seemed repetitious, since by this time in our education, we had so often heard about the importance of protecting the patient, having awareness, and educating the patient about potential safety hazards. We thought we knew everything about legal aspects, and it was all common sense, anyway!

Then we began to read about lawsuits where nurses were held liable for negligence when a patient received injury when a protocol was not correctly followed. Every action undertaken had to have a doctor's order. Even giving an over-the-counter medication, such as aspirin, without an order was considered to be negligence. This class caught our attention.

We found the four days of clinical work to be quite challenging, since we were working a complete eight-hour day in the various nursing departments. We were in the RN role, and our responsibility included caring for a large number of patients at a time. Quite obviously, this was preparation for the real world of work, and an eye opener in time management and setting priorities.

Team leading was the most popular form of hospital nurse management in the '60s. The RN was the team leader. She was responsible to assign patients, give patient reports, and provide detailed patient care instructions to the members of her team. The team usually consisted of the RN, LPN (licensed practical nurse), and a nursing assistant. The RN did not take any patients, but helped the team out as needed, and she communicated patient changes to the physician. All members of the team were to help each other in taking care of assigned patients.

In the interest of patient recovery, communication between team members was priority number one. Changes in patient care were based on the physician order. Following up on those changes was another learning area, as we gained experience in transcribing physician orders. Previously, we had done total care for one patient, now we were learning to care for as many as six to ten patients.

With the reality of working as a "real nurse" came the day in and day out struggle to locate the needed equipment, such as O2 tents. In that era, if a patient required the use of oxygen, a tent was often used. It came from central supply and was basically a large, plastic, clear tent-like device that was connected to an oxygen outlet. The edges of the tent were held in place by tucked-in sheets around the patient. There were no saturation of oxygen (SaO2) monitors to assess lung function, and respiratory therapy was still off into the future.

The patient chart was a cumbersome collection of paper. All patient information from the physician was recorded in the chart, including doctor's orders and patient progress notes. All other departments involved in the patient's care recorded information in the chart. The patient chart included lab reports, x-ray reports, and nurses' notes. In addition, nurses kept a cardex that listed the required needs of the patient. It was used for checking medications, treatments, and lab work, and it must be kept up to date. Finding patient information was readily available using this tool.

In today's hospital world, most patient information, including physician orders, is computerized.

A few classmates had married, much to Miss Barber's dislike, and others had wedding plans in the near future. Most classmates were sending out job applications far and near. Some wished to be "As far away as I can get!" Others planned to stay right where they were for the time being.

It was exciting to plan ahead and think about the future. For those of us still living at home with our parents, we hoped to finally break those strings. Maybe we would make enough money to be able to rent an apartment, or possibly afford to buy a car. We weren't going to miss some things like living in the dorm. But, no longer having the instructor available to help would mean we would have to figure things out on our own. Would we be forever looking things up? Would it take us forever to care for six patients? Would we be able to do it?

In just a little over a month, we'd be graduating. It couldn't come fast enough for most of us! We were ready to move on, listen to The Beatles sing, "I Want to Hold Your Hand," buy a Coke for about fifteen cents and gas at twenty-five cents a gallon. We'd be starting new jobs soon, and we might even make as much as $350 per month. Life was good!

We had to manually roll down the car windows, wind our watches, and get up to change the channel on our black and white TVs. Battery operated everything had not begun as yet. Life was simpler, and we accepted things as they were, never dreaming of all the changes that would occur as have happened in our lifetimes.

Our class, being the first to graduate from this newly formed school, had no school pin to distinguish it from all others. Traditionally, schools of nursing bestow upon their graduates their nursing school pin, and the pin was to be worn as part of the nurse uniform.

A pin designing committee from all three classes within the nursing school had formed. They researched, helped design, and finalized the school pin, using the Methodist Hospital mission statement: Not to be Ministered Unto, But to Minister. To continue the historic Asbury-Methodist tradition, the committee included the anchor from previous Asbury-Methodist nursing school pins. An artist friend of Sue Tingerthal, Yanis (Johnny) Akmentins, designed the outside shape and the stylized anchor for the pin. Bronze, gold, and silver were used to cast the pin. It would be presented at our graduation ceremony.

A committee of classmates joined together to plan details of our graduation ceremony that would occur in four weeks. They chose a style of uniform that all of us would wear. They also chose the songs we would sing. Others in our class were working on our yearbook, the first of the nursing school.

The last four weeks of our education involved practical learning, as well as some social requirements. The nursing service department gave us another "tea," where we were obliged to dress up and behave quite prim and properly.

Another wonderful get-together was an elegant dinner party given by Dr. and Mrs. Hoffert at the Minnekahda Country Club in Minneapolis. We wore our finest clothing, complete with gloves,

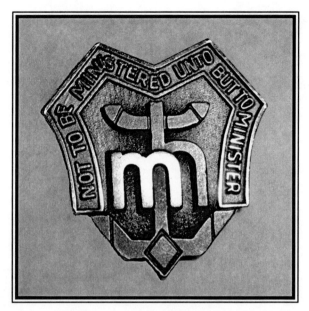

Photo of the Methodist Hospital School of Nursing pin.

stockings, and heels! We were served a lovely dinner, kind words were spoken, and we were given a beautiful, silver-plated, picture frame. Dr. and Mrs. Hoffert had a way of making each of us feel very special.

In that time, when a nurse graduated from an accredited school, she could work as a graduate nurse and basically perform all nursing procedures until receiving the state board results. After testing, it took approximately six weeks to obtain the results. There were five parts to the exam. If a candidate failed any part of the exam, she had to wait three months, with decrease in salary, before being able to retake the failed portion.

After the seemingly endless preparation, June 11, 1964, finally came. We were about to graduate! The ceremony was held at Richfield Methodist Church with the commencement program underway at 8:00 p.m. We all were dressed in the same uniform with three-quarter length sleeves, those white stockings, caps, and our brand new white shoes. Everyone was primping their hair and getting their makeup just right.

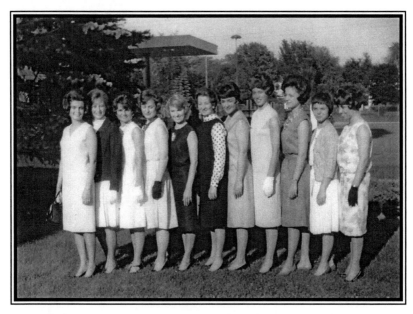

All dressed up for the Minnekahda Club: Barb Carlson, Mary Peterson, Sue Tingerthal, Monyne Jahnke, Sue Lehmeyer, Carolyn Ukura, Sandy Johnson, Vera Kemp, Vicki Lymburner, Linda Mortensbak, and Karen Young.

As we marched into the sanctuary, we each were presented with a lovely bouquet of red roses. The pews were filled with husbands, parents, relatives, boyfriends, friends, and faculty members. The Reverend George W. Chant gave the invocation. Greetings from the medical staff was presented by Dr. Hoffert. Mrs. Shirley Kohlhase from the Alumnae Association gave congratulations. Reverend John B. Oman gave the commencement address. He advised us toward life-long integrity and humility in doing our jobs, and in our lives. His talk was entitled, "It's a Great Time to Be a Registered Nurse."

There were two songs sung by Fred C. Nordstrom. Then it was finally about to happen: the conferring of our diploma and our school pin. Our pin was placed on our uniform by Miss H. Joan Barber, and Mr. Clifford Retherford, of the board of directors, handed each of us our diploma.

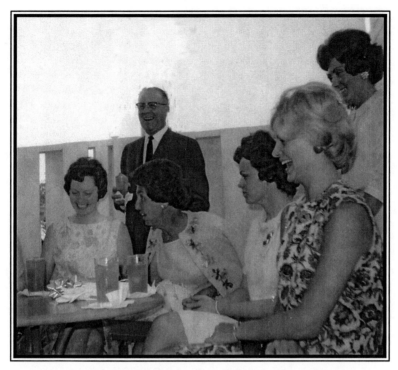

On the patio of the Minnekahda Club: Beth Johnson,
Dr. Hoffert, Mrs. Hoffert, Velma Jean Shelton,
Erma Lobnitz Uglem, and Judy March.

Our hearts were racing! This was it. We were nurses. Our class
sang three selections, "I Believe," "You'll Never Walk Alone," and "I'll
Walk with God." I could see tears in my mother's eyes. I had no tears. I
was so excited and proud to have finished! We strolled out, one by one,
to "Pomp and Circumstance" played by pianist, Margaret Stranger.

The dreaded State Board Exam was to be taken about four
weeks after graduation. That exam had been in the back of our minds
for three years now. It was to be taken over two days time. Each exam
had 150 to 200 questions, and there were five separate exams: medical, surgical, psychiatric, obstetric, and pediatric nursing.

I remember being in a classroom with no air conditioning
at the University of Minnesota in mid-July. The windows were open,

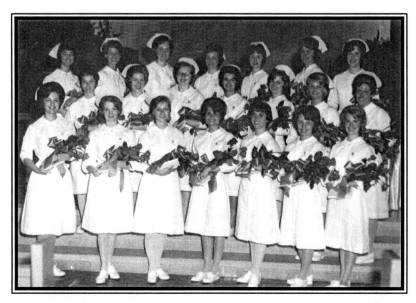

Graduation. Back row (L) to (R): Sandra Johnson, Vera Kemp, Elizabeth Johnson, Velma Jean Shelton, Betty Beard, Judy Mishek, and Karen Velte. Middle row: Linda Mortensbak Gustafson, Jan Kmieciak, Judy Stoneback Rasmussen, Barbara Carlson, Monyne Jahnke, Erma lobnitz Uglem, and Judy March. Front row: Vicki Lymburner, Carolyn Ukura, Mary Peterson, Sue Tingerthal, Karen Young, Sandra Morrow, and Sue Lehmeyer.

and they let in the thick humid breeze of summer. Each test consisted of many multiple-choice questions. Sometimes the question was so long and detailed it seemed like the point of the question was totally lost. It was a big challenge to be undertaking this momentous task. In the end, most all of us passed the state board exam. A few classmates had to retake a portion of the test, but we all finally passed, and we entered the world of work.

And so, our three years of learning about our profession and learning about each other came to a close. We had become a family, always knowing that there was someone in our class we could turn to about our feelings with ease. We no longer were those naïve young teenagers, but we felt we had matured and were well prepared to begin our profession. Only a few of us stayed on at Methodist Hospital to continue our nursing careers.

As we prepared to leave the dorm that final time, we were excited, had tears in our eyes, and wondered if we'd ever be able to live up to Miss Barber's final advice. We said our goodbyes and promised to keep in touch with each other. We had formed a family, and now our family was entering a new phase.

As I look back on our lives fifty years ago, I see us as young, energetic, and confident. Our three-year nursing program had well prepared us to adapt and work in any nursing environment.

THE END OF THE BEGINNINGS

EPILOGUE

I had no idea when we began collaborating on writing this book how time consuming a process it is! I felt strongly, however, that we needed to write our memories about those days. So I began by sitting down, and with pen in hand, I started writing. My mind went back to that September 11, 1961, day when, filled with varying degrees of apprehension, all twenty-two of us came with our belongings to the Methodist Hospital dormitory, a building that was torn down many years ago to make way for an expansion of the hospital.

We started with the first year and continued writing year by year. We accumulated data as memories were sparked by talking with each other. We read what other classmates had written about their experience and researched what was needed for accuracy.

Our education provided us with many job opportunities in the various fields of nursing. Some members of our class relocated to other states, and others moved to different areas in Minnesota, but most continued to work. Some took time off to raise children, and then returned to the nursing world. About a third of us worked in psychiatric nursing; others have worked in acute care hospital settings, public health, and physician's offices. Some worked nurse management in long-term care. Others found themselves in the business world, giving information about health care. Many went on to advance their nursing education and received their bachelor of arts or science degrees. Further, a nurse practitioner license was earned by Sue Lehmeyer Dudding.

I worked as a nursing instructor for twenty-seven years at a community college in Iowa, where I taught a variety of nursing subjects. I taught in the two-year associate degree program, where a huge amount of material was covered in a short time. It was my feeling that these nurses needed at least a six-month internship to get used to the world of work.

When we graduated fifty years ago, we were ready to work and didn't need much tutoring. Today, nursing has become much more complex and challenging, needing ongoing education to keep up. I remember telling my own students that the patients they were taking care of in the hospital were the patients that I cared for in the specialized intensive care unit during my nursing school days. Health care has greatly changed in fifty years.

Our classmates now are scattered. Some we see regularly, others hardly at all. Our accomplished goal has been to have a reunion every five years. Our fiftieth reunion looms on the horizon. We look forward to sharing this work with them.

We have attempted to give the reader a glimpse of what the world of nursing school was like back then.

—Jan Kmieciak Stenson

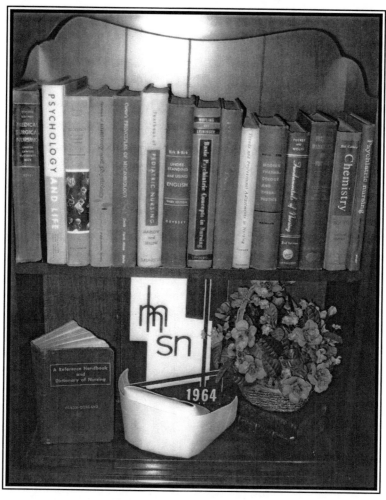

Memories of books, cap, and our 1964 yearbook.
Photo by Karen and Brad Miller, Freeborn, Minnesota, 2013.

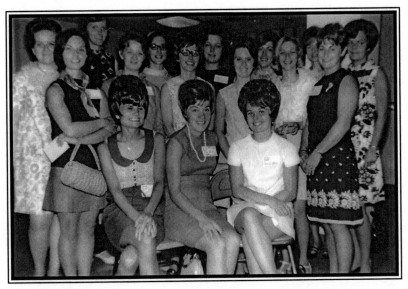

Our five-year reunion in 1969. Standing (L) to (R):
Barbara Wyland, Linda Mortensbak Gustafson, Beth Johnson,
Carolyn Ukura Kuechle, Sandra Johnson Cliff, Karen Young
Miller, Vicki Lymburner, Sue Lehmeyer, Judy March,
Mary Peterson Cady, Betty Beard Welke, Monyne Jahnke Reich,
and Velma Jean Shelton. Sitting: Sue Tingerthal
Jan Kmieciak Stenson, and Sandy Morrow.

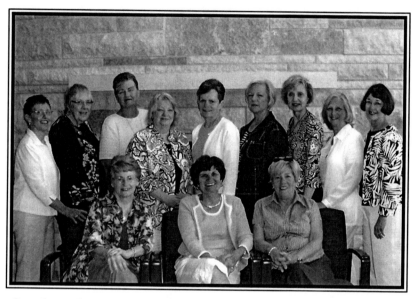

Our forty-five-year reunion at the expanded Methodist Hospital
in 2009. Standing (L) to (R): Karen Young Miller,
Karen Velte Thorson, Judy Mishek Adams,
Carolyn Ukura Kuechle, Velma Jean Shelton,
Vicki Lynburner Thompson, Betty Beard Welke,
Mary Peterson Cady, and Sandra Johnson Cliff Ware.
Sitting: Monyne Jahnke Cotton, Sue Tingerthal Shull,
and Jan Kmieciak Stenson.

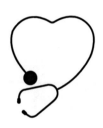

CPSIA information can be obtained at www.ICGtesting.com
Printed in the USA
BVOW03s1202080514

352540BV00002B/5/P